ANOREXIA NERVOSA AND RECOVERY:
A HUNGER FOR MEANING
Karen Way

AN ADVANCE REVIEW

"A highly accessible and readable account of the experience of anorexia nervosa, and particularly, the process of recovery. In contrast with much of the clinical and popular literature, Ms. Way lets the patients speak for themselves, drawing on the depth of interviews she has conducted with recovering individuals. . . . It underscores the fact that recovery from this devastating illness does occur, and holds out a ray of hope to those for whom little seems available. While this book will appeal to a general audience of readers, it should be particularly helpful to those struggling with anorexia and their families."

Richard A. Gordon, PhD
Clinical Psychologist in Private Practice
Red Hook, New York

Anorexia Nervosa
and Recovery
A Hunger for Meaning

HAWORTH Women's Studies
Ellen Cole, PhD and Esther Rothblum, PhD
Senior Co-Editors

New, Recent, and Forthcoming Titles:

When Husbands Come Out of the Closet by Jean Schaar Gochros

Prisoners of Ritual: An Odyssey into Female Genital Circumcision in Africa by Hanny Lightfoot-Klein

Foundations for a Feminist Restructuring of the Academic Disciplines edited by Michele Paludi and Gertrude A. Steuernagel

Hippocrates' Handmaidens: Women Married to Physicians by Esther Nitzberg

Waiting: A Diary of Loss and Hope in Pregnancy by Ellen Judith Reich

God's Country: A Case Against Theocracy by Sandy Rapp

Women and Aging: Celebrating Ourselves by Ruth Raymond Thone

Women's Conflicts About Eating and Sexuality: The Relationship Between Food and Sex by Rosalyn M. Meadow and Lillie Weiss

A Woman's Odyssey into Africa: Tracks Across a Life by Hanny Lightfoot-Klein

Anorexia Nervosa and Recovery: A Hunger for Meaning by Karen Way

Women Murdered by the Men They Loved by Constance A. Bean

Reproductive Hazards in the Workplace: Mending Jobs, Managing Pregnancies by Regina Kenen

Our Choices: Women's Personal Decisions About Abortion by Sumi Hoshiko

Anorexia Nervosa and Recovery
A Hunger for Meaning

Karen Way

Harrington Park Press
An Imprint of The Haworth Press, Inc.
New York • London • Norwood (Australia)

ISBN 0-918393-95-7

Published by

Harrington Park Press, an imprint of The Haworth Press, Inc., 10 Alice Street, Binghamton, NY 13904-1580

Library of Congress Cataloging-in-Publication Data

Way, Karen D.
    Anorexia nervosa and recovery : a hunger for meaning / Karen Way.
      p. cm.
    Includes bibliographical references and index.
    ISBN 0-918393-95-7
    1. Anorexia nervosa—Popular works. I. Title.
RC552.A5W39   1992b
616.85′262—dc20

91-23995
CIP

CONTENTS

Acknowledgements   vii

Introduction   1

Chapter 1: Emptiness   9

Chapter 2: Society's Girl   25

Chapter 3: Families   41

Chapter 4: Onset   55

Chapter 5: Chronicity   69

Chapter 6: Choices   83

Chapter 7: Changes   95

Chapter 8: Meaning   115

Reference Notes   137

Resources   141

Index   143

ABOUT THE AUTHOR

Karen Way, MA, is a writer in Washington, DC, specializing in the social sciences and women's issues. Her understanding of the crisis-of-being wrought by anorexia nervosa is drawn from her own brief bout with a borderline form of the disorder. Way holds an MA in psychology from Goddard College and is a doctoral student in sociology at the American University. She is married to Washington radio personality Cerphe Colwell.

Acknowledgements

Several individuals played significant roles in bringing this project to fruition. I'd like to thank:

• Dr. Ellen Cole, coeditor of Haworth Innovations in Feminist Studies and my first graduate advisor at Goddard College. This book would never have happened without her untiring enthusiasm, encouragement and support.

• Dr. Esther Rothblum, coeditor of Haworth Innovations in Feminist Studies. I'd like to express my deepest gratitude for her belief in this book, for looking beyond the initial rough edges and seeing merit in my work.

• Jeanine Cogan, PhD candidate at the University of Vermont, who read and reread the manuscript at the various stages of the process. Her insights and ideas were invaluable in helping me to sharpen my work.

• Dr. Jeffrey Rubin, my thesis advisor at Goddard, who challenged me to reach for "that next halfstep" beyond what I thought I could accomplish.

• Lisa McGowan, production editor at The Haworth Press, for her sharp eye and constructive input; Eric Roland and Patricia Malone, assistant editors; and everyone at The Haworth Press for doing their jobs so well.

Thanks also to Andrea Lowenstein, Dr. Rolf Kaltenborn, Lisa Baumgardner, Lars Karlsson, Marc Trupp, Jerry Berkow, my mom and dad, and my husband, Cerphe.

Finally, this book would not have been possible without the 21 women who set fear and apprehension aside to share their personal struggles and triumphs in the journey to recover from anorexia nervosa. Thank you for trusting me. I couldn't have done it without you.

Introduction

I didn't plan on studying anorexia nervosa when I started graduate school. In fact, the subject of eating disorders was one of the furthest things from my mind.

Back then I didn't like writing, talking or even thinking about food, weight or eating, because when I was 17, I had a bit of a scare. At the time I started college, I was about 5′6″, maybe 120 pounds. But after a few months of dorm food, desserts at every meal, late night snacks, and many other forms of "stress-eating," I gained the proverbial "Freshman Ten." (Of course, in retrospect, I realize my weight of 130 was normal for my height.)

It seemed that the women in my dorm were obsessed with their weight. Especially my roommate, who was three years older and two inches taller than I. She continually lamented the fact that she was a "huge" six pounds away from 112 — her "ideal" weight. That's all she ever talked about. And next to her, I felt like a real blimp. (Later that year, she dropped out of school to become an NFL cheerleader, but that's another story.)

I was very depressed and lonely, being away from home for the first time, overwhelmed by the pressures and demands of college, especially since I was a year younger than everyone else. Even though I was on an academic scholarship, and objectively, must have shown some promise for scholarly pursuits, I was very insecure and doubted I could cut it. If I failed, I'd disappoint my family and everyone who knew me. It would be so humiliating for the Class of 1980 Valedictorian to flunk out of college. What would people think? I'd be a total failure. It made me unbearably anxious just thinking about it.

My scholarship didn't cover much toward my living expenses. Even with a student loan, I needed extra money for school. That's part of the reason why I was absolutely thrilled when I landed a part-time job at a women's health spa.

As a Spa Assistant, my job was to walk around in a leotard, weigh and measure potential new members, give tours, demonstrate the equipment, and get everyone excited about joining the club, so that someone else could take it from there, sign them up, and make money. My other duty was teaching aerobic dance classes — usually two to three in one evening; four or five on Saturdays.

When things were slow, I worked out and did things like weighing and measuring myself, again and again. Mirrors were everywhere and slowly, but surely, I started getting obsessed.

Since I worked nights, I had to miss dinner at the dorm. But I didn't mind. By the end of the semester, I'd easily dropped my Freshman Ten. And then some.

By February of that year, I weighed in at 116. A lot of the other women in my dorm noticed my weight loss and complimented me on it. They wanted to get jobs at health spas, too.

At that point, I had never felt so triumphant in my life! School and grades no longer seemed much of a concern; how much I weighed was a lot more important. In fact, the first thing I did when I woke up was hop on the scale.

I found it was getting a lot harder to lose weight once I reached 116, but I wanted to desperately. Losing weight was the one thing I had a handle on, the one thing I could succeed at. It was right there in black-and-white, a number on the scale that no one could dispute. Not even me.

But 116 didn't seem good enough anymore. I had this problem — a monumental problem, in my eyes. My inner thighs were "fat," and no matter how much I ran, danced and jumped up and down, the "fat" just wouldn't go away. I focused on my problem intently. It disgusted me.

Clearly — in *my* mind — I could stand to lose a few more pounds. If Kristina, my roommate, was 5'8" and thought 112 was perfect for her, then I had to be at least 106 — three pounds less for each inch of height.

My weight was stubborn at that point. But I was determined. So I buckled right down and cut out nearly everything — everything but **salads, vegetables** and an occasional banana (cut in half, to savor now and later). I even took over-the-counter diet pills. And much to my delight, the weight dropped off.

I stopped having periods around 110. But I didn't care, because *I* was losing weight. *I* was succeeding in a feat heralded as one of the major accomplishments of modern life in our society. As my weight loss continued, I became pompous and arrogant. I felt superior, holier-than-thou, and looked disdainfully at "lesser individuals" who could not achieve what I did, who could not lose weight like I did.

At times, I felt lightheaded; other times, I was in a sort of euphoric fog. I was very difficult to be around, because I was snappy, impatient, impulsive, unpredictable, and very obstinate — especially when others would get on me about what I was eating. Just ask my mother.

In March of 1981, I lost my job at the health spa. I didn't care, because I was going to weigh 106 pounds. And that was *much* more important. But to my disgust, when I reached my goal weight, those insidious thighs were still with me. At least, that's how I saw it: I wasn't quite "there" yet.

Maybe 104 would solve the problem. Then I began wondering what it would be like to be under 100. I rather liked the idea of weighing 98 pounds, and that became my new goal. But before I got there, something happened that jarred me into stopping this process, and perhaps even saved my life.

It was the summer before my eighteenth birthday. I was floundering around at various odd jobs, trying to find something steady that would get me through my sophomore year.

I must have had four or five jobs that summer — at a restaurant, department store, and several aerobic dance studios. Curiously, at each one, I found myself the object of unwanted, often aggressive, male attention. Maybe it was because I looked so frail, weak, and vulnerable, or maybe it was just that I was insecure, unassertive, and had a hard time turning down dates and these men knew it. Perhaps that's why I experienced so much sexual harassment that summer.

This unwanted attention scared me. I didn't know how to stop it and for the first time, I felt that what I had done to myself was very dangerous.

I remember thinking right then and there, "If this is what it means to be thin, then I don't want to be thin." And as strange as it sounds, that's how I shook myself out of anorexia. I was *afraid* to be that thin.

The next year, when I was 18, I gained more than 40 pounds (and as a side note, grew two inches taller). Increasing my size was my way of protecting myself. Curiously, with a few exceptions, I didn't experience much harassment that year, so it seemed that gaining weight offered me safety.

The following year, I met someone who cared a lot more about who I was than what I looked like. For the first time in my life, I felt no pressure to lose weight because he loved me just the way I was. Soon I felt the same way too.

Throughout the next year, as I finished college and got more involved in my work, I began to acknowledge — a bit grudgingly at first — that there were things I did well. Not *perfectly,* as I'd always aimed for before, but *well.* Gradually, as I began to accept more and more of myself, I didn't need a shield of weight to protect me anymore, so I dropped the extra pounds of armor. But most importantly, I began to concentrate my energies on just being me.

For the next several years, I focused my attention on exploring my likes and dislikes, where I was going and what I wanted to do with my life. Rather than only doing things that I thought would please other people and make them happy or proud of me, I began to discover what *I* wanted and what would make *me* happy. For the first time in my life, I was getting to know myself.

It was rough going at first. Rather than knowing what I wanted, what I *didn't* want seemed a lot easier to grasp in the beginning. I explored every avenue that struck my fancy and got involved in all sorts of fun, even a few flaky pursuits that I'd always wanted to.

Slowly but surely, I truly began to know myself and even began to like myself. Suddenly, rather than constantly trying to change myself to look, act or be like someone else or some ideal, I found myself just wanting to be me.

With this newfound self-acceptance, I learned to stand up for myself, fight bullies, and not let other people (individuals, groups, or mass culture) push me around. I learned to define my boundaries and to protest loudly when I felt others were encroaching. Of course, recovery took *a lot* of work — largely through my own introspection and self-study—as well as through connections with others, interpersonal relationships, and short-term counseling.

With this new freedom to simply be me, I learned that freedom and responsibility were closely intertwined—that I was free to do whatever I wanted, as long as I didn't hurt anyone. And when I truly cared about myself, I didn't want to hurt me, either. As I began to make more positive choices for myself, I gradually discovered a calling, a purpose, a meaning in my life.

Somewhere in the midst of this process, I blew the dust off of that once-scary topic of anorexia nervosa and began delving into it once again. Only this time, I had a candle to light my way.

For years, I hadn't known what to make of that "phase" I went through when I was 17. Surely, I couldn't have been anorexic. I mean, no one seemed overly alarmed by my weight loss. I wasn't skeletal. I wasn't shunned by everyone I met. I was just real thin. And I snapped out of it so quickly, with my weight catapulting in the other direction . . . I just didn't know what to think about it. So I tried not to.

In retrospect, I *did* meet the clinical definition of anorexia nervosa: (1) Refusing to maintain a minimal "normal" weight for her* age and height—at least 15% below an acceptable minimum; (2) Being intensely afraid of gaining weight or becoming "fat," even while markedly underweight; (3) Perceiving her weight and body image in extremely distorted ways—insisting she's "fat" when she's emaciated; (4) Experiencing amenorrhea—missing at least three consecutive menstrual periods.[1]

This realization was triggered one night as I paged through one of my psychology textbooks and the words leapt out at me: anorexia nervosa. As I read the text, I grew increasingly annoyed at the condescending, superficial tones of the male authors, who were smug and arrogant in ridiculing the anorexic for her "immature, developmentally-arrested" mind and "crazy" behavior. Moreover, the treatments they advocated—force-feeding, hospitalization, and behavioral therapy (reward-and-punishment models like one would use to train an animal, with solitary confinement for "disobedi-

---

*In view of the fact that 90-95% of all anorexics are female, I am adopting the use of feminine pronouns throughout this book.

ence'')—made me furious. I knew they were wrong—dead wrong. At one time, I'd been there myself, and in my mind, what they were promoting was total idiocy. Although hospitalization *is* necessary in life-threatening cases, it is extremely counterproductive when a program is rooted in behaviorism, i.e., releasing the patient when she has gained a "safe" weight and paying little attention to whether she is emotionally equipped to handle life on the outside. (See Chapter 5 for more on this.)

I felt obligated to set the record straight. Deep down, I had a hunch that my experience and insights could help others. Saving another woman from going through what I did was all the motivation I needed.

To avoid the trap of overgeneralizing through my own experience, I expanded my frame of reference, testing my theories through comprehensive theoretical, then interview research. My primary goal was for others to hear the voices of women—previously silent—to illuminate a crisis-of-being that few truly understand.

Through the course of my research, I interviewed 21 women in the U.S. and Sweden who identified themselves as recovering (or recovered) from anorexia nervosa. I located 16 of my interview subjects through notices placed in the health sections of metropolitan newspapers, four through support group meetings, and one through a personal contact. Six of the women I talked with felt they were fully recovered from anorexia nervosa; the remaining 15 considered themselves to be at various stages of the recovery process.

At the time of the interviews, their ages ranged from 19-44, although the majority were in their mid- to late-20s. Five were students and 16 were professionals—seven of whom held advanced degrees. All socioeconomic backgrounds were represented, although the majority said they were from middle-class households. Three were daughters of alcoholics; four had been raised in single-parent families. Twenty of the women I interviewed were white; one was black.

Except for one interview that I conducted by telephone, I met with each of the women for interviews that ranged from one to four hours in length. We talked in a variety of settings—restaurants, shopping malls, parks, hospitals, their homes, my home, and my office.

Although I had a standard list of questions to refer to, the interviews were conversational in nature — a sharing of struggles as well as triumphs. I tape-recorded and transcribed each interview to form the backbone of this book.

The pseudonyms I use generally correspond to a specific individual, but to protect the identities of the women I spoke with, I changed names and altered or omitted identifying information. The words, however, are their own.

My only hope is that together, we can encourage and inspire individuals who are struggling to recover from anorexia nervosa, and in the process, enlighten friends and family who are simply trying to understand.

Chapter 1

Emptiness

Chelsey answered the door in a white tank top and shorts, struggling to restrain Ginger, her golden retriever, by the collar. As I followed her inside, she apologized profusely for her house "being a mess." I could barely hear what she was saying, but it was immaculate.

Chelsey began struggling with anorexia nervosa two years before, when she was 25. She was a working professional with a graduate degree; married, no children. She described her family background as middle class and traditional—her father worked in sales; her mother was a housewife. The middle daughter of three, Chelsey portrayed herself as "a rebel" in Catholic school, although with time, she settled down, worked hard, and earned her undergraduate and graduate degrees at a local university.

She was very petite—just over five feet tall. Over the phone, she told me she was recovering from anorexia nervosa, but to me, she still looked extremely thin.

I tried to subtly ask Chelsey her current weight. She told me it was 77 pounds. I must have instinctively winced because she quickly assured me, "It's not *that* low."

She searched my face briefly for a nod or other expression of agreement and immediately added, "I eat really often. I just don't eat *meals*. Like I'll have two crackers for breakfast—crackers and tea—saltines or something. For lunch, I usually get a salad. And I have my diet dressing. Or I'll bring my own tuna fish with diet mayonnaise and oat bran or something. So I don't really eat meals, but I'll eat a lot between meals. Not anything *bad*—just crackers or something."

When Chelsey said "crackers," she meant two saltines, 10 calories each. "I keep track of everything I eat and drink *every* day," she remarked with a tinge of pride in her voice. "I've been keeping track of calories for almost two years. Every day. I never miss a day. And I know by heart what [calories] everything has. It's real easy to do now.

"Vegetables are *great!*" Chelsey added brightly. "They hardly have any calories. And seafood is pretty safe. But I don't eat red meat. I eat a lot of chicken. Grilled or something safe. But I never *fry* it, or like, put *sauce* on it. As long as it's skinless and grilled, it's safe. I haven't had anything fried in a *long* time. Well, I *have* had french fries. Like on the weekend. But fried chicken or . . . I don't eat hamburgers. I eat very little bread because I see bread as a waste of calories. They're so *many!* What else . . . anything in a cream sauce. I haven't had a cream sauce in two years. I eat chocolate though. I used to eat 500 calories a day during the week, and if I wanted something chocolate, I'd eat 200 calories the rest of the day so I could have something with chocolate in it for the 300."

To most people, it's mind-boggling that a person could be so engrossed in food, yet only consume 500 calories a day. Most people do not understand how in the world a person could survive on so few calories day after day after day, and not pass out or double over from the constant gnawing pain in the pit of their stomach.

Chelsey would assure you it's easy. "After a while, you really *don't* know when you're hungry and when you're full anymore," she remarked. "I'd always heard that, and I thought, like a few years ago, 'Well how do people *not* know when they're hungry?' But I really feel that now. I could eat at any time — I'd *love* to — but I really don't know what hungry means because . . . I'll get dizzy, I'll get headaches, my stomach will be burning, but I don't see that as hunger. I see that as . . . something else. I know that I'm empty because I haven't eaten. I just don't perceive that as hunger. I think of it more as emptiness, and that feels good, to be clean and pure. And then when you put food into you, you're ruining it. It's going backwards, going in the wrong direction."

In Chelsey's mind, not eating was purifying. To her, starving — fasting — conveyed the underlying symbolism of asceticism. It certainly was not simply dieting for the sake of dieting — nor "dieting gone haywire" — but pursuing the ultimate state of thinness to feel cleaner and more pure — a better, more perfect person.

When I talked with Chelsey, vigilantly guarding against fat was the most important thing in her life. She clung to it desperately. That's why she went to such great lengths to prevent the horrible predicament of "becoming fat."

"If I have a bad day, or retain too much water, I might, like, go over," Chelsey said, as a point of illustration, "so I have to be *a little under*, just in case. Or if I'm going on vacation, then I have to lose three pounds before, so I can even out, so I can eat while I'm away. But then I still can't. I still go crazy worrying about everything anyway."

Chelsey wasn't always like this. "I never used to be a perfectionist," she admitted, "but that came with this. In fact, in high school, I didn't do that well. I was pretty rebellious as a teenager. I was in trouble a lot. And I think that's part of this, too, that I didn't like who I was then, so I'm trying to go back and make up for it. Now I have to be totally perfect at everything. Now I *am* a perfectionist in a lot of ways. If I do something, it has to be perfect or it really bothers me.

"Sometimes I'll torture myself," Chelsey continued, "especially if I feel like I have to punish myself. I'll walk through a bakery and I won't let myself get anything. It's like, *smell* it, and then walk out. Or I'll walk down the candy aisle and look at all the things I want. Like if I screw up something, then I don't like myself and I'll punish myself — make myself walk up the candy aisle and not be able to get anything."

Consequently, along with the underlying symbolism of thinness meaning purity, cleanliness, and goodness, to Chelsey, denying herself food also served as a form of punishment — discipline — for "screwing something up," for bad behavior. Tempting herself in the way she described *could* be a way of "torturing" herself — to see how strong she was, mind over body. Sometimes she'd just be angry. That's why she'd do it; that's why she'd want to punish herself.

For instance, if people would tell her she looked "good," Chelsey starved herself even more strenuously in order to punish herself because she wasn't thin enough. "When people say you look good," she explained, "it's like they want you to look fat. If they say, 'Oh you look good,' then I think, 'Well, I must be getting fat.' I don't want to look good to *them* because that means that I'm not too thin anymore."

On the surface, it may not make a whole lot of sense, yet, the anorexic hates herself so intensely that she'll twist every situation — subjectively distort it — just to make sure she'll always end up losing, always failing. In her mind, she's not good enough to win. She's not worthy. Once entrenched in this framework, she's convinced she never will be.

Chelsey said she compares herself to everyone. "If I see someone who's obviously thinner than me, I get real mad," she confessed. "If I go out to dinner, and I'm feeling okay because I know I'm thin, and then someone walks in who's really skinny, I just don't want to eat. It ruins my whole night.

"I look at everybody now," she continued, giving me a quick once-over. "I'm always asking my husband, 'Is she thinner than me?' It drives him crazy. He'll say, 'I'm not even going to answer that.' But I really have trouble with being able to tell, I think."

"Most of the people I know, I weigh less than, so it doesn't matter what they weigh, as long as I weigh less," Chelsey remarked with a slight laugh. "*I* felt really good when I could go into the preteen department and get my shorts. I thought that was *great!* Because I was in there with all these 12-year-olds and I felt like one of them, you know? I thought, 'This is really weird. I'm 27, why do I want to be 12?'"

Chelsey confessed that her husband had a hard time dealing with her anorexia. "He doesn't really understand that much," she said. "A few months ago, when my doctor wanted to put me in the hospital — I really didn't think it was necessary — my husband jumped on that bandwagon and he kept talking about it — I think because he didn't know how else to deal with it. Until about six months ago, he never really said anything about it. And then all of a sudden, it became a big issue. I don't know why. And he started on me about what I was eating — 'Well you can't have that, that's not enough for dinner! You have to eat more or you're going to go to the hospital!' And he was constantly asking me what I weighed. He got to be a real nag about it," she concluded with a laugh. "He's gotten a *little* better, because I told him that it makes it more difficult to pressure me. But it was really annoying for a while." Not to mention, pointless. At this stage, there's really nothing he — or anyone — can do to change Chelsey's mind.

When I spoke with Chelsey, losing weight was the only thing that really mattered — that meant *anything* to her. And to give that up, to lose *that*, she was convinced, would be like losing a part of herself. "If I don't focus on that, then what else, . . ." she trailed off. "I have a really busy life — it's not like I have nothing to do — but it seems like it's the most gratifying. And if I don't focus on that, what am I going to focus on that will give me this much gratification?"

When I met Jenny, she 'had just come in from a run. She struck me as a friendly, happy-go-lucky college kid, or so it seemed.

At 19, Jenny had been slipping in and out of anorexia for four years. She had never been hospitalized. "I was right on the border, but they said no," she told me. "Three more pounds and I would have been. And that would have been awful! They intravenously feed you, and you don't know *what* they're feeding you . . ." she trailed off.

I soon realized that *that* was the scariest thing to Jenny about anorexia nervosa — being hospitalized and having any semblance of control she thought she had taken away from her. Once we started talking, I began to suspect that she rather liked being anorexic. Even though she told me over the phone she was recovering, I had my doubts that she really wanted to. In fact, her energies seemed to be very much invested in staying right on the border, at 5'3" and 95 pounds. Not quite low enough to be hospitalized, yet just low enough for others to notice the problem and treat her for it.

"I see a therapist once a week," Jenny said flatly. "My parents are always asking me, 'Would you like to see her twice a week? Is any of this helping?'"

"It really isn't," she admitted with a sly grin. "My parents talked with my therapist last Christmas and she suggested I start seeing a nutritionist, someone who would tell me what to eat."

"So . . . I started going to a nutritionist," Jenny remarked smiling. "I see her about once a month and she just weighs me. I don't use any scales. I hate numbers. I'm not getting obsessed with numbers again because when I started my last diet, I was dropping a pound a day, and I'd get depressed. I don't deal with numbers. I just go by the way I look and feel and how my clothes fit, that kind of stuff. And so I get weighed in and she gives me an exchange diet, something like Weight Watchers, except I'm supposed to eat *12* milks and *13* meats and so many fats. I like that, because then I can eat *what* I want, *when* I want it.''

"But you know,'' she confessed, "I like *skim* milk. I'm not going to drink whole milk with more calories and stuff like that. But she's really nice and she specializes in people with eating disorders. Like everybody who sees these psychiatrists gets sent to her.''

"She's gotten me up to 2,500 calories a day,'' Jenny added. "I used to be at 2,100, but now that I've been hovering around 89, 90, she's given me a boost. I told her, 'I'm sorry, but I do not find time in the day to consume 2,500 calories. I'd have to get up at 3 o'clock in the morning and go to bed at 1 o'clock at the end of the day in order to eat that many calories.' And she said, 'Well how about six mini-meals?' Well, I'm in classes with 13 people and if I'm going to pull out all of this food and say something like, 'I'm hypoglycemic; I have to eat it,' it's just embarrassing. I find it embarrassing. I find it embarrassing to always be eating. Maybe it *is* a carrot stick, maybe it *is* nonfat yogurt, but I'm eating, and people are watching me, and I feel uncomfortable.''

"Now I work every day,'' Jenny added, "and I work in an office that's real open and the refrigerator is there, and every time you go there, everything jingles and jangles. People see you, people hear you, you know? And okay, it would be different if I weighed 400 pounds and I was going to the refrigerator every 13 minutes. But I can't block that out of my head. I still think people are watching me every single time I go, so . . . I do not find enough time in the day, and I tell her that.

"She [nutritionist] has me keeping a food diary, so I write down everything I eat every day, and the portions. But I always overestimate,'' Jenny confessed with a grin. "I just want *a little bit*! A little bit is fine with me. I don't want a big *gob* of cheese, I just want a little bit. If I eat a gob, I'm going to get sick, and I'm going to get a lot of cholesterol and calories.''

Jenny's powerful resistance to weight gain was abundantly clear. "I haven't put on weight in over a year," she admitted. "I don't know what's there, what's holding me back and why I just can't get over. They say a normal weight for me is 110-115, and when I think about when I weighed 115 pounds in 10th grade, I was *fat*. You know, *maybe* if I had gone to the gym and toned it up, it would have looked better, but when I think about that number, I just can't. I refuse! And I've got to get over that. I mean, 115, I'll probably look good, I'll have a chest, the guys will be running, that'll be great, you know? But right now, I look at myself and I say I'm skinny. I look at myself and I'm fragile, but I get so much feedback from other people, 'Oh, you're just small, you're not skinny.'"

Being judged as "on the borderline" seemed to bother Jenny a little bit. It made her angry when people didn't believe she was anorexic, no matter how hard she tried to convince them. "I just got this new roommate in January, and I didn't tell her until last month that I went home every Thursday to see a psychiatrist, and she said, 'You have an eating disorder? I just thought you were really small. You look fine to me.'

"There are so many mixed messages," Jenny continued. "I'm trying to get through this, and then there's this whole society that's on a diet, and I'm fighting them because I'm eating all of this food and everyone else is like, 'Well, I'll just have this and this cracker.' My roommate, she's a maniac. She rides a stationary bike about 20 miles a day. She's always walking around doing something. She's got to be standing because she's burning more calories standing up than sitting down. And I have to *live* with this!"

By contrast, Jenny felt her own exercise routine was quite reasonable. "I don't racewalk like an idiot," she assured me. "I just walk *fast*. Because running hurts my knees and my ankles and I just don't like that jarring, because there's lots of curbs around here. But I can do about five miles an hour—that's about a mile every 12 minutes—and I move. I *move*. I want to feel my heart pounding, I want to feel like I've gotten a workout."

"I'm totally addicted to exercise. I can't stop," she confessed. "I always feel that everybody's better than me and so *I* have to be better. I was just talking to my psychiatrist about the exercise, and I said, 'They say three times a week, 20 minutes is fine, that will keep you physically fit. But I'm sorry, I've got to be better than everybody. I'm going to do an hour a day. I don't care. That's good for *me*.'"

"When you get so obsessed with it," Jenny concluded, "spending a hundred dollars every three months on Nike Airs doesn't matter. As long as you're skinny. As long as you're getting your exercise. I don't know, exercise didn't seem that important when I was in high school. But now, it's *really* important."

Jenny revealed that she's not comparing herself with anyone else, but to an absolute standard of perfection. "I compete with myself," she told me. "What *I* can do the best, what *I* have done. And with grades, well, I got two B's the last time, I'm going to get one this time. It's always this inner competition, like I'm trying to prove something to myself, I'm trying to prove something to my family, to my friends. And it's really kind of stupid."

Like most women struggling with anorexia, Jenny expressed some difficulty in knowing when to stop, in knowing when how much was too much. "Especially with the number of things I take on," she remarked, "I'm just a whirlwind."

When we spoke, Jenny was on her summer break and told me she felt incredibly lazy. "This six weeks, I'm not doing anything, just going to work," she said. "That's all I'm doing. I work over on campus and if they give me a bunch of paperwork, I have to sit for six hours, and then I feel guilty about eating dinner. I feel guilty that my thighs are turning to fat all day long. I'm getting secretary's butt, you know? And I just feel incredibly lazy. I'm not doing anything. My mind is not working; I'm not in a class. What the hell am I doing? On the weekends, I'm just going to the pool. Sitting there for three hours. My thighs are getting fat. I'm not doing anything. I'm baking myself, giving myself skin cancer. That stresses me. It stresses me. I think, 'Oh God, maybe I should walk an extra hour Saturday morning because I'm going to be at the pool.'

"And then every time I go into my nutritionist," Jenny complained, "if I lose a pound or a half a pound, she'll say, 'Well what do you want to do now?' And I say, 'Why don't you just give me a magic pill that will put on five pounds kind of slow.' Because I get so sick of eating food. I'm supposed to eat *so much* every day, and I'm just not used to it. It gets disgusting, because I'll only eat certain foods. I mean, I eat pizza and ice cream, but then if I *do* eat that, then I feel bad and I say, 'I have to be good for a week because that cheese is, you know, affecting me in my arteries.'

"The food is the control," Jenny admitted. "My psychiatrist always asks me, 'What would you think about if you didn't think about food all day?' I don't know. School, but that's really boring. Boys, but I don't have one in my life. My family, but they really kind of bore me. My friends, what am I going to do this weekend. Errands. But food is my mainstay and that's the little high that I'm on. I'm still on it and it still possesses my life. I have fun with it. It's my little thing. It's my toy; it's my game; it's *mine* – don't take it away!"

Anorexia nervosa fills the emptiness, and after a while, it's very clear that there's no room for anything else. "If I go into my therapist and start crying or whatever, she'll ask, 'Well what are you feeling?'" Jenny remarked. "And a lot of times, *I don't know*. I'll just start crying and I don't understand. I'll start talking about my family, or even food, about how frustrating it is . . . . A lot of times, I don't *know* what the feelings are. I may have experienced them, but I've shut them out for so long that it's really hard to get in touch with them and know what they are. Is this depression? Is this sadness? Is this happiness? Is this anger? What is this and where is it coming from? Is it other people, or is it within me?"

One of the most difficult dilemmas for Jenny is that there's nowhere to run. No matter where she goes, no matter what she does, she is constantly reminded of the supreme importance of thinness in our society.

"I can't go through a day without somebody mentioning food or weight," Jenny remarked bitterly. "Everybody talks about it. It's on my mind every day. If I try not to think about it, somebody else brings it up. It's just society! Our entire society is obsessed with food, weight and thinness!"

Not surprisingly, Jenny is having an extremely difficult time casting all those messages aside and finding her place, finding a balance. "The biggest question I have," Jenny said, "is what is a normal eater? What person doesn't think about food? I can't even grasp it because it's so weird to me. Because I've been so wrapped up in it for so many years. What does [such] a person think? Like guys — they don't think, they just eat whatever they want. It totally just kills me and baffles me. I do not understand how people eat like that — eat normally. Don't worry about it. Even people that pack their lunch, they have to think about what they're going to pack. Everybody's got to think about it every day, but people not to get obsessed with it . . . . I know absolutely not one person that does not do that. So I've got to find that person and talk to them.

"I hope to get the answer sometime," Jenny added softly, "what it's like. Because I don't eat when I'm hungry anymore and it's going to be really hard to start to understand that signal again when I get up to my maintenance [healthy weight]. What does it mean to be hungry? What does it mean to eat at a time that's not scheduled? It's going to be a real big thing, because I haven't listened to my body and eaten in response to it since the 9th grade. I don't know what it's going to be like to eat like that and stop when I'm full. What does that mean? I don't know. Because I've always starved myself."

Yvette was a bit apprehensive when we first spoke on the phone. We talked at great length before she finally agreed to meet in a safe, neutral location.

When I first met Yvette, I was struck by how muscular she was, despite her extreme thinness. She spoke thoughtfully and deliberately; her mannerisms and facial expressions were reminiscent of a child's. "I've thought about this a lot," Yvette opened, "you wouldn't believe, because I am very introspective, and I believe, I'm convinced, I *know* that my family is extraordinarily dysfunctional, *extraordinarily*. And I wanted to tell you one thing about this," she added, "I have never told *anyone* [that I was suffering from anorexia nervosa]. Anyone. I've never told anyone. I've never told my parents, I've never told *anybody*. And that just blows my mind that I've had this experience that I've never *dared* to share. But after I talked with you on the phone, I knew I had nothing to fear. So I wasn't afraid.

"All of my sisters, we're *all* crazy," Yvette continued with a laugh. "We are, we are! And I think that we're all paying the piper. I think that the eating thing is, in my case anyway, not the core thing. It's almost incidental. It was my coping mechanism for being in a family where I had no other coping mechanisms. I had no control. None. But I could control that.''

"You should see my home!" she suddenly exclaimed. "I'm 37, and my home is absolutely, totally spotless! You could come in and you could eat on the bathroom floor! It's *perfect*! I mean, I am compulsively organized. But I'm controlling my world, you know? This is *my* space, *my* world, *mine*! And I can't stop it. I've thought about it, 'Try stopping it,' but I *can't*!''

"I'm terrible without structured time," she admitted. "Everything's got to be organized. I have a list, everything's on a list. I write a list every day and I follow the list. Everything. I'm *very* organized. Loose time is not good.''

It quickly became evident that total control was the key issue in Yvette's life. "I know I look sort of loose and easy now," Yvette remarked, "but when I go to work, I am *perfect*. I mean, I wear good clothes, I do my makeup well, and I'm very aware of my appearance. I must look at my mirror 20 times during the day to make sure it's absolutely right. I'm very conscious of my appearance. And it's important to me, because it's my *self*—it's a source of self-esteem for me to look good. I think I have very low self-esteem, so when I know I look good, it reinforces the self-esteem that I *do* have. That's why I'm so neat and organized. Because *that* is my control. It's like I can't get it from the inside, so I get it from the outside. That's what I do—I get all my feeling good about myself from the world around me. Because I don't feel good inside.''

Yvette confessed that she had a hard time forming personal relationships. "I tend to be extremely isolated," she told me. "There's absolutely no one in my life. Zero! I'm *very* solitary. I don't think that I am happy with that, but I'm very afraid. I don't want to be exposed, and I don't want to be hurt, and I'm very protective of myself because I've been hurt *a lot*. And I just don't want to do that. I want to cope with the world on my own terms, you know? And I know I'm losing out on things that way, I know I am, but I'm very aware of that and I'm paying that price. At times, I *do* get lonely, but I'm paying that price. I know that. And sometimes, I get a little scared, because I think, 'Well I'm 37—if it's this way now, what's it going to be like when I'm 47?'

"I'm very rigid," Yvette continued. "I'm five-foot-nine, and I like being 110, I like weighing 110, and I like weighing 110 *every day*. And I don't eat *anything* that's not good for me. I *never* have sugar — *ever*! I haven't in years. I never have anything — *anything* — that's not good for me. I'm very vegetarian and I don't eat a lot. I really don't. I just eat what I need. And I know how many calories I eat. I know exactly what I did. When I'm doing things, I don't think about food, but I know exactly what I'm eating. Always. I'm very aware of nutrition and what is going into my mouth. And I *never* eat anything that's not good for me. I'm very rigid. I don't eat unless I really want to. I like being thin. And empty, too.

"But some days," Yvette said in a hushed voice, "even now — even now — say I'll have a big meal or something, and I'll just go like this [holding her abdomen] and it will just hit me, and I'll go in, and I won't even try, I'll just go, 'tshuuuu,' and it just comes right out. It [vomiting] just *happens* to me," Yvette said innocently, as she tried in vain to camouflage her denial. "And I don't feel guilty about it, because it wasn't intentional. It just doesn't want to be there. Even now. Today. It happens to me.

"I don't menstruate," Yvette continued in a detached voice. "I haven't menstruated, well naturally, since 1978. I take estrogen replacement therapy, which is critical, because of osteoporosis and stuff. I don't know whether it's my body weight or the fact that I don't have any fat. Because I'm in good shape. And I think if I would stop working out, I would probably menstruate.

"I feel that my working out — I know for a fact — is my therapy," Yvette added solemnly. "And has been for *years* and *years*. I've been a swimmer since 1974 and I do, oh, two and a half miles a day easily. And I'm also a runner. I run very early in the morning before no one else is awake. And I think that while I'm working out, that is my meditation time. It's *very* important to me," she whispered. "I would rather be *dead* than not have that. That's all there is, as far as I'm concerned. It's a real quality of life."

The center of Yvette's life is controlling everything she eats and exercising religiously. "I get up *very* early," she said, "around four. I get up early. Then I really greet the dawn and I go through a series of stretches, and I jog two miles, and then I swim. Then I go to work. And I work pretty well.

"I do that every day," Yvette said proudly. "You can see why I have a solitary life, because I have all these other things, and my day is crammed. It's really crammed. By being crammed with activity and being so busy, I fulfill myself, you know? And I think there's a certain blindness in that, which I'm very aware of. I blind out the need to be sociable, because I have all these other things that I'm busy doing, you know?"

I wondered if Yvette was happy with her life, with herself. "I don't know if I'm happy with myself," she responded. "I don't know whether I'm a happy person or not. I'm happy if I work out. I'm happy if I do my list. If I do my list, I'm happy. If I don't do my list, I'm not happy."

I asked her if she felt she was in touch with her feelings. "Do *you* think I'm in touch with my feelings?" Yvette asked. "I don't know. I really don't. I try to know, but I don't. I think feelings, a lot of the time, are what you label them as. I think that the stuff is the same, really. I mean, I don't think that feelings . . . I think that anger is different from joy, but I think it's on the same dimension, you know? And a lot of what you feel is what you label it as. I think. I think that, really. I think I feel a lot of numbness, I do. I can be very good at denying things. I think, I *think* anyway, that I can appear to someone to be extremely calm, quiet, and fine — everything's fine — and inside I'm a tempest. So I don't think I'm very good at pinpointing what it is. Nooooo! I think that feelings are almost like something that other people experience."

Anorexia nervosa is an addiction like any other, only thinness is the obsession and losing weight is the fix. When you're anorexic, watching the numbers go down on the scale is the only thing in the world that matters to you. It's the center of your life, the only meaning to your existence.

Pursuing it takes up all of your time, all of your energy. Once the obsession takes hold, no tactics seem too extreme or off-limits. You'll do anything — lie, cheat, pretend, sneak, and deny — to keep the weight loss going . . . to fill the emptiness in your life.

According to researchers Paul E. Garfinkel and David M. Garner (1982),[1] and Donald M. Schwartz, Michael G. Thompson, and Craig L. Johnson (1982),[2] the causes of anorexia nervosa are multi-determined, resulting from a complex interaction of factors within the individual, family, and society.

It's important to realize, however, that the precise influence of familial or societal factors may vary dramatically from woman to woman. Thus, each case must be examined and understood individually. In other words, although the resulting jigsaw puzzle of anorexia nervosa may appear to be the same, the nature of each contributing factor — or each puzzle piece — must be thoughtfully examined in the context of each woman's experience.

There is one common thread linking the lives of all women who succumb to anorexia nervosa, however. Women who become anorexic initially turn to the strategy of weight loss to feel some semblance of control in the face of tragedy, to cope with pressures and demands that are intensely overwhelming — whether it's the death of a loved one, prolonged sexual abuse, a professional crisis, geographical move, or losing a best friend. The particular trigger may vary markedly, depending on the woman's stage in life and personal experience.

As is the case with any other addiction, low self-esteem lies at the core of anorexia nervosa. In *Women & Self-Esteem,* Linda Tschirhart Sanford and Mary Ellen Donovan point out that low self-esteem is common among women in our society, due largely to the universal experience of "female oppression in a male-dominated society." They observe that low self-esteem is the root of many psychological problems among women. Thus, even when an anorexic changes surface behaviors by eating again, the issue of low self-esteem must be addressed and dealt with, or the same addictive tendencies will manifest in other forms and only allow the "one-down" female oppression to continue.[3]

The major issue of recovery, and the key theme of this book, is the necessity of developing a healthy sense of self-esteem, moving beyond the emptiness, and finding meaning and fulfillment in life.

The issue of self-esteem is extremely complex in the case of the anorexic. Her precarious sense of self is fused with an intense perfectionism, which viciously undercuts any bit of esteem she *does* manage to garner. Since she measures herself in every arena of her life — in her appearance, grades, and professional achievements — against an absolute standard of perfection, she never feels "good enough," which only compounds and intensifies her feelings of worthlessness and inadequacy. She is convinced that no one will accept her, approve of her, or love her unless she is absolutely perfect. And to her, for whatever reasons she may have — whether perceived from her family, peers, the mass media, or popular culture — extreme thinness *means* perfect.

The anorexic diets, in a desperate attempt to prove herself worthy, acceptable, and "good enough" — perhaps to her family, the world-at-large, and lastly, to herself. As she focuses on this task of dieting with single-minded conviction, losing weight is a snap.

Consequently, initial weight loss produces profound feelings of euphoria. *She* decided to lose weight and *she* did it herself! She made the needle register a lower and lower weight on the scale, and no one else can take credit for it. *She* controlled that.

Losing weight, particularly in a society such as ours in which "successful" dieting is heralded as a monumental feat, is positively exhilarating to an anorexic! She feels *good* about herself, often, for the first time in her life. This achievement — which everyone can see, which is evident by the numbers on the scale, which no one can deny — is the most powerful and fulfilling experience of her life! Only she doesn't want it to stop, because losing weight boosts her fragile self-esteem. It's the greatest thing she's ever done. She wants to keep it going, to keep losing weight, so she can continue to feel successful and good about herself, instead of worthless and inadequate, like she used to feel.

When an anorexic woman reaches her initial weight goal, she tells herself that she's not quite finished, she's not quite "there" yet. She just needs to lose *a little bit more*. Then, she tells herself, she will be "acceptable" to herself and others, once and for all.

She becomes addicted to this fleeting sense of esteem, to the "good" feelings that this weight loss produces — to this process that she and she alone is in control of, that makes her feel better about herself than anything in the world. So, she continues to lose.

Watching the numbers go down on the scale every day becomes a sort of high for the anorexic. It's what she most looks forward to every morning when she wakes up: how much less she will weigh when she steps on the scale, as soon as her feet hit the floor.

Losing weight makes her feel triumphant — in complete control of her body—and her life. That power, that control, means more than anything else in the world to her . . . which is why she is obsessed with continuing—no matter what the cost.

As her weight plummets lower and lower, an anorexic's mind becomes her staunchest ally. When she examines her naked body in the mirror, she does not see how thin she is. She does not see her sharply-defined rib cage, nor her jutting hipbones, nor the stiff ligaments of her knees, nor the stark outline of her skeleton and her skull, which is so clear and so abhorrent to everyone else. She sees only "fat"—the hips, thighs and buttocks that she has to lose in order to be acceptable.

She subconsciously distorts her body image so she can continue to achieve, so she can continue to feel successful and "good" about herself, with one clear, conscious goal securely in mind: if she loses enough weight, she will reach the coveted, ultimate state of thinness. And then, finally, she will be acceptable and approved of. Finally, she will be worthy of being loved—by herself, and the world at large. Someday. But someday never comes.

Food and weight obsessions envelop the anorexic, engulfing the totality of her existence. There's no room for anything else. There's no allowance—no time, no space—for feelings, for questions, for uncertainties, for "gray areas." Losing weight is the only thing that matters. Everything else in her life is secondary. It's black-and-white, as simple as that. Anorexia nervosa becomes fused with her identity. It's the center of her world. The only thing that means *anything* to her.

Anorexia nervosa fills the emptiness in her life.

Chapter 2

Society's Girl

Some time ago, I was trying to explain to a male friend what it was like for me, growing up female in America.

As a preschooler, I remember staring wide-eyed at the beautiful, glamorous, reed-thin models on the covers of magazines while I waited with my mother in the supermarket checkout line. I studied the cover girl mannequins; I looked up at my mother. Those women weren't like Mother. They wore beautiful clothes, exotic makeup, and windswept hairstyles. They were chic and glamorous. They were very, very thin.

I was sure they led thrilling and exciting lives, like the svelte heroines I watched on my favorite television shows, like the lean, long-legged beauties who seemed to be having so much fun, stylishly puffing cigarettes on billboards while my mother drove by in the car.

It was 1967, 1968. I wasn't even old enough for school in those days, but I remember those images vividly. They comprised my earliest education of what a woman "should be": a flawless face and very, very, thin body. (And it's a sad commentary that those idealized images haven't faded into oblivion today.)

When I was growing up, the "woman as body/woman as object" message was reinforced everywhere around me, on billboards and magazines — even in the commercials that interrupted my Saturday morning cartoons. Being an impressionable little girl, I picked it up in a snap.

As a girl, I learned that I was supposed to be pretty, frilly, and feminine. I was supposed to wear lacy, pink ruffled dresses, bake treats in my Suzy Homemaker oven, shun sports, Tonka trucks, snakes, and dirt, and spend hours on end, gleefully playing with

Malibu Barbie, her omnipresent boyfriend Malibu Ken, the house, the furniture, and the sports car convertible.

.In those days, before the women's movement heightened the awareness that the minds of youngsters needed to be protected from the patriarchal whims of advertising and media executives, the media succeeded quite readily in brainwashing me. But I wasn't the only one. My friends were all exposed to the same message I was: that the role of a woman in our society was to be stunningly beautiful and very, very thin — a man's trophy. That, we were told, was a woman's carte blanche for life. Those who were successful in achieving this feminine ideal were promised glamorous lives just like Malibu Barbie's, or so we were led to believe.

As I described these early memories to my friend, he became increasingly defensive and argumentative at the notion that I was blaming the media — blaming *the media,* mind you! — for our society's obsession with extremely thin women.

He was quick to argue that men are subjected to societal ideals as well. When he was a boy in the 1950s, he told me, the predominant message directed toward him and his male peers was that men must be strong, muscular, and powerful, à la Mr. Universe, Charles Atlas, and football linebackers.

As a boy, he argued, he was also subjected to the calculated ploys of advertisers and the mass media, and was always sensitive to the fact that he was tall and thin and didn't fit the brawny, rugged build of "the male ideal." He spoke of bodybuilding ads in the backs of comic books that he read as a boy, with headlines that read, "Is the Bully Kicking Sand in Your Face?" And the prescribed solution in the copy below the ad: to bulk up like Mr. Universe.

"Okay, then," I challenged my friend, who is still as tall and thin as ever, "why didn't *you* become obsessed with bodybuilding?"

Because, he answered matter-of-factly, he could see plenty of male role models who didn't look like Charles Atlas, yet were still "successful" by all accounts of the word (i.e., who still managed to "get the girl"). He was surrounded by popular actors, singers, comedians, television journalists — even athletes — who were not Incredible Hulks, but still "acceptable" and very "successful." He quickly realized that torturing himself to conform to this male ideal was unnecessary. He knew he didn't have to look like Superman to be "acceptable" or "successful" as a man.

Therein lies the real difference between the role models young boys and young girls are exposed to. Even today, boys are surrounded by a diverse collection of male role models, from rock stars like Mick Jagger, Sting, Prince, and Bruce Springsteen; to comedians like Eddie Murphy, Johnny Carson, and David Letterman; to actors like Bruce Willis, Jack Nicholson, Al Pacino, and Marlon Brando; to television news personalities like Dan Rather and Bryant Gumbel; to financiers and politicians and on and on and on. As these examples illustrate, men are not judged first and foremost by their looks, their body, or their "thinness quotients," but by their talents, their competence, their power.

Yet ponder Western society's most worshipped and popular female "role models." Consider our hottest rock stars, actresses, and fashion models — Madonna, Julia Roberts, Whitney Houston, Jamie Lee Curtis, Paulina Porizkova — not to mention the frivolous category of women who are merely affiliated with famous men — the Marla Maples, Fawn Hall, and Jessica Hahn types. Curious, isn't it, that there is no category of male parallels?

The number of idealized females who are not stunningly beautiful, who do not epitomize our society's obsession with extreme slenderness, who do not conform to our society's relentless feminine ideal, can be counted on one hand. Those who do not fit this ideal, like Roseanne Arnold, Delta Burke, Oprah Winfrey, and sometimes, Elizabeth Taylor, are ridiculed for their irreverent and slovenly "lack of control" — for embodying the greatest of sins in our society — "FAT!" — in screaming tabloid headlines run over unflattering photos, week after week, year after year.

What kind of message does this send to young girls, the brightest minds of our next generation, to our future? That extreme thinness and beauty are essential for a woman to be "acceptable" and "successful" in our society (but not for a man).

It's a message that is reinforced everywhere — on television, billboards, and magazines; by families, peers, and society-at-large. Tragically, this all too pervasive message stressing the dire necessity of thinness, dieting, and weight control is hitting home at younger and younger ages.

Alison, a recovering anorexic who was obese as a child, was only six when the taunting began. "I did get a lot of teasing from the other kids for being overweight," she recalls, "and that was always one of the things that cut right through.

"I can remember being really young," Alison adds softly, "and looking at those ads for Slim-Fast, where they show the 'before' and 'after.' I used to look at the 'befores' and think, 'Oh, if only I could look like the other one, if I could go through this program or that one, then I could be accepted and liked.'"

Chiara, who like Alison, began dieting as a preteen, also endured cruel and cutting remarks about her weight from her peers and says that it greatly influenced her initial decision to diet. "Kids used to tease me sometimes because I was taller, and they would associate that with being fat," Chiara remembers. "I really wasn't. But when I hit puberty, I started to put on some weight, just because of the normal changes, and so kids would call me names. I started young, too — I was 11 or 12. So I started to put on a little weight — I wasn't obese and I wasn't fat, it was just normal puberty. But I got signals from that. Peer pressure contributed to a lot of it."

The seed is planted at a very early age. In fact, researchers Susan and Orland Wooley (1979) find that "anti-fat" attitudes and negative stereotypes associated with being overweight are pervasive even among young children. However, they report that by adolescence, females are affected much more by this prejudicial climate than males.[1]

Jenny remembers it well. "Back in sixth grade, my girlfriends used to talk about being fat and how awful it was, and what size jeans we wore," she says. "We had this one girl, Tami, who had a really big butt and we always made fun of her. That was sixth grade. Back. Back a long time.

"Those were just the little things," Jenny adds. "It got stronger in eighth grade. And then into high school, it just climbed and climbed and climbed. Then we were competing for the boys. And 'skinny is best.' It was a message that was stressed all the way back from sixth grade — just the competition with your friends and everybody. 'Skinny is best.' And you'd see Weight Watchers and commercials on health clubs with Victoria Principal on there looking wonderful. You'd just see it. And you'd want it."

A key element of anorexia nervosa is relentlessly seeking approval and acceptance from others. For many females, males are the "others."

In our male-dominated society, as mass media and popular culture parade the quintessential female image most appealing to men as thinness, even children pick up the message. It's reflected in their attitudes and behaviors, especially at school.

"All thin girls were the most popular," Chelsey recalls. "I don't know if it just worked out that way or what. But I just always liked the way thin people looked. They always seemed to me to be really in control of themselves and on top of everything. Like the fatter the people were, the more out-of-control they were — I just saw the two as being sort of related."

Again, we see that even among young teenagers, the drive to conform to a feminine ideal of thinness to attract male attention — to please males, to "get the guy" — is everywhere.

"My high school was real competitive for guys and all that," Jenny explains, "who was the prettiest, who was the skinniest, and all that kind of stuff. And there was this one girl in school — Jacqueline — who I just envied. Jacqueline was a size three. Jacqueline was dating a senior when she was a freshman. Jacqueline was getting the guys — because Jacqueline was a size three. Jacqueline was skinny. Jacqueline was pretty. And I was going to be Jacqueline.

"She was my goal. I wanted to be Jacqueline," Jenny remembers. "And it was the weirdest thing, because I was a size five, and then I was a three, and then threes were falling off of me. And then, I couldn't figure out why it wasn't working — why I wasn't, all of a sudden, pretty and popular like Jacqueline."

Women are socialized to believe, through mass media and popular culture, that thinness will solve all problems. Like Jenny says, it will make us "pretty and popular." All we have to do is be thin and we'll live happily ever after.

Researchers Paul E. Garfinkel and David M. Garner (1982) point out that the media capitalize and thrive on keeping the magnificent package of thinness alive. They note that the glamorous, beautiful, and successful heroines on TV and films are invariably thin. No surprise, then, that audiences associate thinness with desirability and success.[2]

"All the actresses . . . they are slim," Monica remarks. "And if they are a bit heavy in the beginning, and they realize they are going up in their careers, they diet. So you see them some months later and they are slim. Then you realize if you want success, you have to be slim. You see that on TV. You see it with pop stars, too. I've seen so many starting off as normal, and then going down to real skinny—like Madonna.

"The newspapers and magazines, the movie stars played a big role for me," Monica adds. "I thought, 'Okay, I'm not perfect in my face, so I have to be perfect in my body.' I looked in all the newspapers and fashion magazines. I was very young, I was ten or something—and they told me I have to be very thin, because that's the only way to compensate, to look good in your body."

Why do so many women feel an overwhelming need to "look good?" Perhaps because "looking good" is the focal point for most women.

Brenda, who became anorexic in her mid-twenties, observes, "A man can be overweight but still think he's okay as a person. He separates himself from his body. But for a woman, you *are* your body."

One would think that in the 1990s, as "acceptable" roles for women have expanded to include impressive achievement mandates, the majority of us would base our identities on what we do rather than what we look like. Yet appearance, beauty, and thinness are still at the center of many women's identities.

It's not our fault, however. Entire industries are based on breeding body insecurity in women, as author Susie Orbach (1986) points out. Whether it's responding to the call of beauty editors, diet gurus, color consultants, fashion designers, personal trainers, and celebrity exercise videos; cosmetic counters, tanning salons, aerobic dance studios, and plastic surgeons who will nip and tuck and vacuum all the cellulite away, women are taught to believe they aren't "good enough" as they are. Orbach hints at the "profound alienation" many women have, both with and within our bodies.[3]

Robin, whose weight was below average *before* she began dieting, remarks, "To me I was always overweight, but to everyone else, I was at a normal weight for my height. I got the message from our society that I was too big, in every kind of way — in magazines and on television. When I went into the stores, all the nicer outfits were for smaller sizes. I felt bad about myself, that I was too heavy. I thought it would make a difference if I were thinner. I was looking for external changes to make me feel better."

Women are taught to hate themselves, to hate their bodies. If a poll conducted by *Glamour* magazine in the mid-1980s is any indication, many have learned it quite well. Researcher Marlene Boskind-White (1985) reports that in February 1984, *Glamour* magazine surveyed 33,000 women about their perceptions of their weight and body image. Nearly 75% of the respondents felt they were too fat, even though, by conservative standards, only 25% percent were heavier than they "should have been" and 30% were actually below the norm for their heights. A clear majority also stated they were either "dissatisfied" or "ashamed of" their stomach, hips, thighs, and buttocks. Boskind-White reports the surveyors observed a "steadily growing cultural bias — almost no woman, of whatever size, feels she's thin enough."[4]

Over the last several decades, dieting has proven to be a white-hot topic, a mainstay in women's magazines. Researchers Paul E. Garfinkel and David M. Garner (1982) reviewed the five most popular women's magazines from 1959 to 1978, counting the number of diet articles in each magazine. In the 1960s, there were, on average, 15.6 diet articles published each year; in the 1970s, it shot up to 22.9. They conclude that their findings clearly document increasing societal pressure for women to lose weight.[5]

This pressure is tragically clear in the voice of Heidi. "I remember I could see bruises on my hipbone and up my spine from doing situps and pushups," she says. "I remember I was getting into smaller and smaller and smaller clothes. And I also remember that I could see everything that I wanted to get rid of on my body.

"I didn't see myself as fat, but I don't think I saw what I looked like," Heidi says. "I remember seeing that my face had no color in it. The ball at the end of my nose had gone even. I remember seeing that my eyes looked larger and my cheekbones were sharper and wondering, 'I've got big eyes and cheekbones and a small nose now. Why aren't I beautiful?'"

Since beauty ideals are forever changing—becoming thinner and thinner, and thinner, in the last 20 to 25 years—they're impossible to attain, even with great genes. With so much pressure and focus on appearance, it only causes a woman's self-esteem to plummet.

I believe this intense societal pressure goes a long way in explaining the dramatic surge in reported cases of anorexia nervosa over the last two decades. It occurs on a grand scale for women, who are continually assaulted by the message from every direction—the mass media, peers, families, and popular culture: you must be thin to be acceptable, to be worthy of love, to be beautiful. Not living up to the ever-changing ideal of femininity leads to a lowered sense of self for many women, who feel defeated and "not good enough," for not measuring up to the ideal.

"I think thinness helps in being attractive," remarks Jessica. "Now I have a cousin who's overweight—and she's beautiful in the face—but I think that's one of her drawbacks, why she doesn't date as much. It's because people are so superficial. She's a wonderful girl, but she *is* heavy. She's beautiful in the face, and I just . . . I look at people like that and think about it, and I don't want it to happen to me.

"I'm not saying that being skinny is going to make me pretty, because my facial looks aren't going to change," Jessica adds, "but it may help to get that second look from a guy, you know? And it's not that I'm looking for someone . . . it's just that I want to be noticed."

The "right" appearance will get a woman noticed. That's what women learn, that's what they see. Many women believe that resembling the glorified ideal of the day will make a woman "acceptable," as Nancy illustrates.

"Back when I was in college, Twiggy was very, very popular," Nancy remarks. "And I remember people commenting on the fact that she was very, very thin. When I was in college, I was thin, and my roommate's father would always make comments about my figure, and other people would comment that I was 'nice and thin.' So I always had that in the back of my mind — that thinness was good."

Not surprisingly, Nancy married a man who also bought into this message. "My husband always had this thing about overweight being really bad," Nancy explains. "He always liked thin women. His sister-in-law was very overweight, and he was always making comments and things about her, or he would make comments about other fat women, and so on. So I think I also had it in the back of my mind about that, too — that I would never get overweight for him either."

Nancy learned that dieting and weight control were essential in "keeping her man." The thing was, as each year passed, it got harder and harder for her to embody the ideal image. For as researchers David M. Garner, Paul E. Garfinkel, Donald M. Schwartz, and Michael G. Thompson (Garfinkel and Garner 1982) report, the feminine body ideal has been whittled away over the years, becoming smaller and smaller, thinner and thinner. Through their study of *Playboy* centerfolds and Miss America pageants for the years 1958-1979, they report that the comparison and contrast of the *Playboy* Playmate of the Month's bust, waist, and hip measurements signify "a trend toward a more 'tubular' or androgynous body form." Further, in the case of Miss America pageant contestants, those who captured the crown were on average, five to seven pounds thinner than the average contestant — a trend particularly noticeable over the decade 1969-1979. At the same time, however, these researchers cite actuarial statistics to indicate that the average female under age 30 did, in fact, become *heavier* over this same period of time. This, they note, illustrates the profound tension between the "dream" and the reality — the feminine thinness ideal, in sharp contrast to what women actually weigh — and helps explain the striking preoccupation with dieting and weight control in society today.[6]

In my mind, women's magazines are a chief culprit in perpetuating the preoccupation with dieting and weight control. With flashy covers that glamorize rail-thin models and articles and advertisements that plant and fester the seeds of insecurity, telling a woman that she must continually change and improve herself to be "acceptable," is it any wonder that low self-esteem and self-hatred are such significant issues among contemporary women?

"I've always thought that women in magazines had perfect bodies in these ads, and I wanted to look like them," remarks Chelsey. "I wanted to be perfect. I never had a weight problem—I was always average, never overweight—but I always wanted to be thin. Ever since I was little, I always admired women who were really skinny. I thought they were perfect."

Similarly, Nikki believes magazine advertising played a major role in convincing her that her body was "too fat," that she needed to diet. "I always had this idea that I wanted to be perfect, and to be perfect, I had to be real thin—a ballerina or a model. I was always reading magazine articles about losing weight. I would study models and compare myself to them. Then you always had your friends, too, in the summertime, when bathing suit time came. You'd all have the same conversations. I thought if I followed this particular diet, or that one, it would work. I read all the magazines."

When women are young (and sometimes even when they're not), impressionable, and struggling to figure out who they are, to find their place in the world, these glamorized images that tell women "you just don't measure up" are very cutting, cruel, and hurtful.

"You get very much influenced by the newspapers and fashion magazines, and all of society thinks you should be thin," remarks Helena. "You see all of these photo models, and everywhere the message is saying if you are thin, then you are good."

Jenny prides herself in reading all the magazines—"*Cosmo, Glamour,* you know." "And there was a thing in *Cosmo* about being voluptuous—you know, 'a few extra pounds don't matter; stop killing yourself to exercise and diet; just let it go; men like it,' and stuff like that. But that's *bullshit*! Because you see all the pictures of these skinny people, and *that's* what everybody wants to look like."

Even if women refuse to buy magazines, the glamorous, sexy, reed-thin images loom from billboards, newsstands, and television. There's no escape.

"I was more elitist in what I read," Heidi says with a slight laugh. "But you're surrounded by women's magazines anyway. You don't have to read them to get the message."

You *don't* have to read them. The covers alone convey everything you need to know, and that was enough for Chiara. "I was never one to look through *Cosmo* or *Vogue* because I thought I would never fit that," she says. "But I think I saw a society where thin people always seemed to be appreciated more — even in my own household. I felt pressured by society to be thin. Then my clothes would fit me like they fit the models — the thin people — and people would look at me the way they looked at them."

Images are not the only issue, however. A most unfortunate trend has developed over the last fifteen years. The portrayal of anorexia nervosa has, on numerous occasions, bordered on a sort of morbid glamorization in the popular press and media.

The first example occurred in the mid-1970s, when an article in *Playgirl* labeled anorexics "Golden Girls." Then in 1978, Hilde Bruch's widely-read book, *The Golden Cage*, opened with a description of anorexia nervosa as "a disease that selectively befalls the young, rich, and beautiful . . . affecting the daughters of well-to-do, educated, and successful families."[7]

"Golden Girls"? "Young, rich, and beautiful"? This idea of anorexia being a chic, glamorous, and "desirable" category to be in, hasn't been hindered by all the media attention devoted to the Karen Carpenter story, Cherry Boone O'Neill, Susan Dey, Joey Heatherton, and intermittent media hoopla surrounding Princess Di.

Of course, the glamour, the affluence, the status of anorexia is only a stereotype. Over the last fifteen years, the skyrocketing number of reported cases of anorexia nervosa has permeated all age groups, economic levels, and ethnic backgrounds.

Until the late 1970s, anorexia nervosa was practically unheard of, and consequently, was rarely reported in the media. Before that time, anorexia nervosa was rarely seen; it was an unusual coping strategy that an adolescent female seemingly arrived at on her own. But no longer. Today, anorexia nervosa is not the mysterious, unknown entity it once was. Even the average male is able to utter "Karen Carpenter" in response to the one word cue, "anorexia."

Anorexia nervosa is found everywhere today. Most of the women I talked with had known of other anorexics in school, and observed anorexics in shopping malls, health clubs, or running down the street. With special made-for-TV movies, books and articles devoted to the subject, many women learned all about anorexia nervosa, prior to the onset of their own struggles.

This leads me to ponder a controversial, yet critical issue: could media attention have contributed to the dramatic surge in reported cases of anorexia nervosa over the last two decades? A casual remark by Nancy makes me wonder.

"A couple of girls have said that they got the idea to starve themselves," Nancy says, "from a movie or from a book or a magazine article." That hits home.

The first time I remember hearing about anorexia nervosa was when I saw *The Best Little Girl in the World,* (Steven Levenkron's best-selling book which was made into a TV movie). I remember thinking that the whole concept of anorexia nervosa was rather intriguing — a unique sort of thing to do — because it required so much discipline and hard work to deny yourself the pleasures of eating. I don't believe that I was consciously imitating what I saw when I began losing weight, but I know the movie made quite an impression on me.

Heidi had a surprisingly similar experience. "I first heard about anorexia nervosa when I found the book, *The Best Little Girl in the World* when I was about 13," she recalls. "And I looked at it, and I thought, 'My God, how *stupid*! That could never, ever happen to me.' Those were the exact words that went through my head. And I didn't really think about it again until the last stages, when I got very, very caught up in it."

That causes me to wonder . . . could sensationalized, bordering on glamorous portrayals of anorexia nervosa by Western media lead some females to conclude that anorexia nervosa is *desirable*? Could the continuing escalation in reported cases of anorexia nervosa be partially explained by the "copy cat" syndrome? Is it possible that reading, watching and hearing about anorexia nervosa could plant the idea in a young woman's head and even offer techniques on how to starve herself?

The implications of this premise are terribly frightening. As Western media, pop stars, movies, and other entertainment are exported en masse around the world, even Third World countries are being exposed to Western beauty ideals. This socialized emphasis on thinness is translating into cases of anorexia among females of all ages, ethnic groups, and socioeconomic levels.

Researcher Richard A. Gordon (1990) reports that until the 1980s, anorexia nervosa was rarely seen among blacks or American Hispanics. He attributes the recent shift to increasing assimilation of Western society's dominant cultural values—feminine thinness, achievement, and upward mobility—among many ethnic groups. Gordon cites two cases to illustrate this point: a Black African who developed anorexia nervosa after attending an English university, and a study of female Egyptian college students who exhibited eating-disordered behaviors after studying at a London university. Thus, Gordon concludes, when non-Western groups are exposed to Western values, they become increasingly vulnerable to disorders such as anorexia nervosa.[8]

Researcher Felicia Romeo (1983) reports that anorexia nervosa is rapidly increasing in countries that share Western values of feminine thinness and achievement, such as Western Europe, Scandinavia, Japan, and Australia. As women in less industrialized countries are exposed to Western cultural values—i.e., the glorification of feminine thinness—through exported television, movies, and magazines, the trend will likely continue.[9]

Curiously, however, though the number of reported cases of anorexia has increased dramatically, the proportion of females to males has remained constant. But why? Why are 90-95% of all anorexics women? As detailed earlier, women are socialized to define themselves primarily through their appearances. In addition, there are extreme pressures on women of all ages to conform to ever-changing beauty ideals in order to be "acceptable" and worthy of love. Yet there's another key factor that merits attention in explaining both "why women?" and "what has changed in the last twenty years to explain the surge in cases of anorexia?"

Quite simply, I believe it's the metamorphosis of the "Superwoman" ideal of femininity. I honestly don't remember how or when it happened. It must have been somewhere between *That Girl* and *Mary Tyler Moore* that the Superwoman Bride of Frankenstein was created. Or maybe when Helen Gurley Brown took over *Cosmo* and began indoctrinating susceptible minds around the world with the "Having It All" myth: women are supposed to do it all, be it all, have it all — a thrill-a-minute career, a dashing knight in shining armor, great sex, a chic wardrobe, tastefully decorated home, and above all, a very, very thin body beautiful.

Sometimes I feel sorry for those women who grew up and came of age in the 1960s, 1970s, and 1980s, who have weathered a positively schizophrenic combination of confused messages. As little girls, the doctrine was to be "sugar and spice and everything nice," then all of a sudden, the message changed midstream. Suddenly, Malibu Barbie had a career. And women of all ages were supposed to, too . . . . to know what they wanted to "be" — something substantial, exciting, exotic, and impressive.

All of a sudden, women were instructed to dress for success in a man-tailored neutral suit, white blouse and floppy scarf-tie (for that dash of color). Women were supposed to achieve and compete. Those who had grown up with Barbie and Ken, cultivating essentially empty lives, suddenly felt the rug had been pulled out from under them.

"I felt pressured to have a career, but I never really knew what I wanted to do," remarks Jessica. "I had a hard time deciding. I didn't want to go to college. I just needed time, I think. It would have done me a world of good if I had just worked out of high school for a while, and decided on something from there, instead of having all the pressure, 'You've got to go on; you've got to know exactly where you're going in life and what you want to do.'"

Researcher Richard Gordon (1990) notes that the radical cultural changes witnessed since the late 1960s have resulted in many vulnerable women "becoming caught in the uncertainties and ambiguities of a drastically altered set of expectations," and hence, to anorexia nervosa.[10] Not only are women "supposed" to be pretty, frilly, and feminine (as always), but tacked on are new role requirements of achievement and career success. It's causing unbearable anxiety, pressure, and stress for many women.

"I think that today, it's harder to live than it was forty years ago," says Helena. "It's harder in many ways, and I think that's why many women are becoming anorexic when they are older. When you're 30 or 40, it is also a stage when you can be thinking, 'What am I doing [with my life]?' And you have so many feelings inside that you have to keep them down, and so you starve yourself or eat only a little bit of food, because you feel pressure and anxiety and want to cope somehow.''

Through starving and relentlessly focusing on exercise and losing weight, anorexics can block it all out — all the pressures, the anxieties, the pain.

''I felt a lot of pressure, because I thought, 'How am I going to do all this?'' Chelsey remarks. ''How am I going to be married and work full time and have kids?' It's so much to try to do — and do it all *well*.

''You get to the point where it's so much that you withdraw,'' Chelsey concludes. ''You can't do it all perfectly, so you're not even going to think about it. You just focus on . . . this other thing.''

Yes, anorexia nervosa offers an escape. Anorexic women are so wrapped up in coaxing that number down on the scale that there's no room for anything else. No anxieties, no pressures. Then they don't feel the pain. They don't feel anything at all.

Chapter 3

Families

Twenty-five-year-old Kelly was barely seven years old when she realized the tremendous importance of thinness in her family. It was the first time she witnessed the ridicule, pain, and rejection that one suffered in her family as a result of being overweight. The memory scarred her life permanently.

Seven-year-old Kelly woke up one morning to find a curious sheet of paper attached to the side of the refrigerator. On it were three columns, labeled "M," "D," and "J," and underneath the letters were five three-digit numbers. To Kelly, it looked sort of like a puzzle, like the numbers she added on her arithmetic worksheets at school.

As she stood on tiptoe in her nightgown and pink fuzzy slippers, carefully studying the cryptic letters and numbers, it suddenly dawned on her that "M," "D," and "J" stood for Mom, Dad, and Julie, her sister. "I thought they were playing some sort of game," she recalls with a wry smile, "and wondered why *I* wasn't invited to play."

Kelly felt left out. She *never* got to do the grown-up things that Julie (who was all of 11 years old) got to do. Being the middle child, Kelly was *always* second. Julie was the first to do everything!

Suddenly she heard her parents laughing in another part of the house. Julie's voice grew even louder, as her shouts echoed down the hall. The commotion moved closer as "M," "D," and "J" headed toward the kitchen. Kelly scurried back to the breakfast table, bewildered and confused about what was going on.

Her mother, father, and sister crowded around the puzzling sheet of paper on the refrigerator. Her dad laughed gleefully as he penciled numbers in each column and Julie cried uncontrollably.

"The numbers were pounds," Kelly explains, "their starting weights followed by what they weighed each morning after. See, my mom, my dad, and my sister were competing against one another in a family weight loss contest."

That morning, Kelly's parents had both lost weight—which Kelly quickly learned was a coveted measure of esteem and respect in her family. But her sister Julie had gained three pounds. For that, her parents—most specifically, her father—taunted and ridiculed Julie for her "lack of control" and accused her of "sneaking cookies" and "being a pig."

"I suddenly wasn't very hungry," Kelly remembers, with tears in her eyes. "It was a real turning point in my childhood. That morning when I was seven years old, I learned that no matter what else happened, I could never, ever, EVER be fat. Because then my parents would laugh at me and make fun of me, just like they did with Julie and then they wouldn't love me."

Kelly's story brings to mind a powerful point that is typically overlooked in the examination of family factors that make a young woman vulnerable to anorexia nervosa: Families may play a major role in parroting and reinforcing the obsession with thinness as a feminine ideal.

As in Kelly's case, sometimes it's not so subtle. In fact, many women recall hearing their parents scorning and ridiculing overweight family members and making meanspirited and cutting remarks about acquaintances or strangers on the street they labeled as "fat" when they were growing up. Some observed the vigilance with which their mothers, sisters, grandmothers and aunts guarded against the most devastating of all predicaments—extra poundage—with the on-again, off-again crash diets, the powdered drink mixes for breakfast and lunch, the low-cal frozen entrees for dinner and saccharin-laden sodas in between; the talk, talk, talk—about pounds gained, pounds lost, calories in this and calories in that. The curious way fathers, brothers, uncles and grandfathers acknowledged and responded to thin women—their approving remarks and glances, the way they would "size a woman up," as if a woman's measurements are the first and only things their critical eyes see.

Consequently, the message that filters down to a young girl is clear and unmistakable—that in her family, being thin is of the utmost importance in gaining acceptance, respect, and approval. That her parents—and the world at large—will love her only if she is thin.

Most of the women I talked with described growing up in family environments in which weight control was a major issue. Twenty-year-old Nikki, who virtually stopped eating when she was 14 years old, says she first became aware of the all-encompassing importance of weight control when she was eight.

"At that time, my sister and my mother were going to diet workshops," Nikki remembers. "My mom had a weight problem and my sister was beginning to, so a schoolteacher suggested that my mother take my sister to diet workshops before it got to be a real problem in adolescence."

At the tender age of eight, Nikki was initiated into the grown-up world of weight control. "I grew up thinking that's what women do—they go on diets," she says. "My mom was constantly trying to lose weight or flatten her stomach, as was my older sister. I thought that dieting was just part of being a woman."

Consequently, it was no surprise several years later, when Nikki began going through puberty, that she was determined to correct her "weight gain problem." "When I started to get chubby, I got very paranoid," she says. "My sister at that time was a problem child, and so I equated fat with being a rotten person. I equated being thin with having friends and decided I was going to be thin and popular. I was determined to be everything my sister wasn't. I was going to be friendly, successful, happy, popular, and *thin*. So I started toting around a calorie book at school and became very calorie-conscious."

Nikki was mimicking the behaviors she'd learned were part of being a woman—vigilantly guarding against the most perilous of evils—"fat." And so began Nikki's spiraling descent—lower and lower and lower, until she finally collapsed and was hospitalized at 77 pounds.

Clearly, an extremely weight-conscious household encourages a young girl's preoccupation with thinness for acceptance and approval. Growing up in such a family, her perceptions of the supreme importance of a thin body are grossly distorted, as slenderness is worshipped and glorified as the key to her happiness and success.

In fact, for Jenny, it was a classic case of learning-by-observation. She picked up the monumental importance of being thin simply by watching the anguished attempts of her mother relentlessly striving for it.

"My mom has been dieting for as long as I can remember," Jenny explains. "She's been on everything—Weight Watchers, NutriSystem, Diet Center. You name it, she's been on it. She did really well on the last diet—she lost about 120 pounds." The maximum her mother weighed was 250 or 260. "She's about 5'4"—big bones, but she's short and stocky, like my sister."

Naturally thin, Jenny wasn't *too* concerned about her own weight until the 9th grade, when she began attending a competitive private high school with her older sister. "In 9th grade, people would say to me, 'Your sister's FAT!' And so all of a sudden, I began to classify her as fat."

The uneasiness quickly set in as Jenny began mulling over the scenario in her head. "Sister and Mother are both fat. Father is skinny," she recalls. "I began wondering, 'What's going to happen to me? Well, I'm a girl. Mother and Sister are fat. I'm going to be fat.'"

To Jenny, feedback from her peers, coupled with the emphasis on weight control in her household (her father was a distance runner and weight conscious as well), prompted her to closely monitor every calorie she consumed to guard against the contemptible outcome.

As with Nikki, dieting was perceived as a rite-of-passage for Jenny. Throughout her childhood, Jenny had been well-versed in the necessities of dieting that were all wrapped up in being a woman. And now it was her turn to carry on the family tradition.

"My mom had all these diet books around the house," Jenny explains. "Even as a kid, I used to read the diet articles in magazines. I grew up looking at this stuff—seeing it, hearing it. And then I would read the magazines. You're reading *Glamour* in sixth grade and it's, 'Do this diet, lose ten pounds in this many days.' I started reading about the recipes and getting all these low-calorie ideas. I started making dinner every night because I didn't trust what my parents were making for me because *I* was on a diet and I needed my diet food."

Chiara also grew up in a family that worshipped thinness. "My mother was always overweight and she was always on diets, *constantly* on diets," Chiara explains. "My middle sister was always petite and small, and everyone kind of looked after her, because she was so 'fragile.' I used to be a little jealous. Because I was taller for my age than the other kids, I always looked bigger and I hated that. My sister looked smaller and seemed to get all the attention. Then there was my mother with all these talks about diets. And on her side of the family, a lot of them are overweight, so whenever I would be around them, I'd look around and panic, 'Am *I* going to be like that?'"

This was a common theme among the women I talked with. Monica, who became anorexic at age 12, found the weight control message was strongly stressed in her household as well. "My mother is very obsessed with weight," she says. "She was a little bit too heavy when she was young, and now she is thin and thinks it's very important . . . because she likes to dress nicely and to look as a woman 'should' be."

Yvette also notes her mother's concern with weight. "My mother was always very weight conscious—she weighed herself every day," she says. "She's a very tall woman, about 5'11"—and always weighed 143 pounds—which sounds like a lot, but on her, was very thin. And she's still very food aware. In her letters, she'll write about food—like what she fixed for dinner. She's always thinking and talking about food."

For many women I talked with, the preoccupation with dieting and thinness seems to be somewhat of a tradition, carried down through the generations.

"My mother was a ballet dancer, so she had to be thin, of course," says Helena. "And also my grandmother, she behaves as if she has anorexia. So I perceived the message from my family always, that you had to be thin. If I wouldn't be thin, I wouldn't be good.

"My mother and three sisters have very small bones—really, really small bones and *my* bones are more like my father's, so I couldn't be as thin," Helena adds. "But when I was getting thinner, all of my thoughts were, 'Oh then I will satisfy my mother.' So it was very much for her . . . I thought that if I were really thin, she would want to . . . love me.''

For many women, thinness was one way to earn the love and approval of Mom and Dad. Yet many women remember it was Dad who first hit the compulsory dieting/weight control message home. It was reflected more in Daddy's eyes: that in order to earn acknowledgement, approval, and love, "his little girl" couldn't be anything but thin.

Yvette remembers it well. "When I was 13, I was just getting a little plump, and my father came home, and he said, 'You're getting fat,'" she says. "I remember not eating for almost a month. I would take my food and wrap it up in a napkin and put it under the table. All I wanted was to please my father.''

Like the majority of men who have grown up in Western societies, Yvette's father was extremely appearance-oriented, which Yvette perceived as a condition in earning his love. "I can remember talking to him very sincerely, and he would interrupt our conversation and say, 'Stop frowning.' He wasn't even listening to what I was saying,'' she remembers. "He was just looking at me, sizing me up, evaluating my appearance. I can remember coming home from college and sitting at the table and watching the news (we watched television while we had dinner) and I remember looking at the television and just sitting there. I couldn't do anything. I was like a robot because all I was thinking about was how I appeared from my father's point of view. And I went through that for years — for *years*!''

For some women I talked with, other conditions were tied to the externally-based, appearance-oriented mandate. For example, that they would earn approval and love *only* if they achieved and accomplished great things.

Jill, who became anorexic soon after she dropped out of college at 19, felt this achievement pressure intensely. "I know for my dad, a lot of what's important is based on externals — inside stuff, too, but it's harder for him and I to communicate that,'' Jill explains. "It's not as common as, 'Oh, you look good today — that's a pretty dress. Oh, you look great; you got a suntan. Oh, your hair looks pretty.' He's more apt to say *that* than, 'Gosh, it's fun to be with you; you're such an insightful person. It's fun to be with you; I like what you talk about.' Being a businessperson, he's not used to saying those kinds of things.

"Now if I came home and said, 'I just completed this project and I feel so good and I made this much money,' he'd say, 'Wow, let's talk about it!' He can relate to that," Jill says. "When I became an adolescent, I started identifying being [achievement-oriented] like my father, to get my father's acceptance. But he's a workaholic, so I never made that bond."

Yvette felt a strong achievement mandate, as well, in addition to other conditions that had to be met to earn her father's love. "I got the message that I needed to achieve from my father," she explains. "My older sister and my younger sister were both very good singers. We're a very musical family, but I didn't sing as well as my sisters, and my father made that very clear—that I was not as good as the others. And as a consequence, I thought, 'What can I do? I can do well at school.' So I became very good at school, and I did that for a long time. I wanted my father to be proud of me."

Succeeding in school was one surefire way to earn parental acknowledgment and approval for many women. Yet some felt extreme pressure, believing they had to truly excel—to be perfect—in order to be worthy of love.

In families, there is often intense competition between siblings in the desperate struggle for attention, acceptance, and love. When a daughter doesn't feel "as good as the others" in music, sports, or math—when she doesn't feel she could possibly measure up—her self-esteem suffers a barrage of hard-hitting blows.

"My sisters and my brothers had no problems in school. They were straight-A students and really didn't have to work hard at it," says Jessica. "I had a comprehension problem and took remedial reading. I struggled for my C's, and every time I came home with what *I* thought were good grades, my father would always come back with, 'Well, what's wrong with a B?' Or, 'Now that we've got this accomplished, let's work on something else.' But it never seemed to be enough.

"I really wanted to please my father," Jessica adds. "I don't know why. I consider myself . . . . I'm the spitting image of my father. The others are my mom. And Dad doesn't show outward love very well, so it was real hard to get in his graces. No matter what I did, it just never seemed to be the right thing. I felt so alone, because I just didn't have what my sisters had. They've both completed college. I've never completed a four-year college. I never even got a bachelor's degree. My brother's got a master's even. I'm just tagging along at my own little pace and never reaching what they did.''

Needless to say, relentless sibling comparisons can lower a girl's self-esteem. Chelsey, who has an older and a younger sister, still berates herself for "not measuring up" to her sisters' accomplishments and is plagued by feelings of inferiority and inadequacy.

"I competed with my older sister, but she was so much smarter than me," says Chelsey. "I always felt that she was so much better than me and I still do. My older sister is a surgeon and my younger sister wants to be. And they're both brilliant; they've always gotten straight A's. Everything they do is perfect. They never fail in anything. I was always the dumb one. I mean, my father never came right out and said it, but it was sort of understood.

"I never felt I was good enough, or that I was something my parents could be proud of, that they could brag to their friends about," Chelsey adds. "When I got my master's I felt like I'd accomplished something. But even then, it was no big deal—it wasn't like I got an MD or anything.

"My mother was very into us getting a good education, but not as much as my dad," Chelsey explains. "We had a lot of pressure on us to succeed, to achieve. We went to a private school and there was a lot of pressure, especially with my father. He always wanted us to do more and more.''

This perception was one I heard over and over again. Although, as I'll discuss later, the family histories and backgrounds of the women I talked with varied dramatically, all shared a common theme: They grew up believing that absolute standards for achievement and appearance were conditions that had to be met in order to secure the acceptance, approval, and love of significant others.

This message of conditional love was by no means relegated only to fathers. "My mom really stressed the achievement message," says Nikki. "She really wanted to have perfect children to show everyone she was the perfect mom. She didn't feel successful. Even though she had a college degree, she quit her job because she wanted to be the perfect housewife.''

Nikki resented her mother's apparent focus on external achievements, because to Nikki, it was ''selfishly motivated, as if having 'perfect children' would show the world that she was a 'perfect mother.' My mother was always telling me, 'Well you have to have a college degree, you have to have your own career, and you have to be independent,' but *she* didn't do that. I always wondered, 'Why is this something that *I* have to do, but you didn't do it?''

When the ''Superwoman'' ideal is stressed within the family, it creates an exorbitant amount of pressure on a young girl, who's got enough on her hands simply trying to survive adolescence. When a girl perceives her family embracing sociocultural mandates of appearance, thinness, achievement, and success as an anthology of conditions that *have* to be met in order to earn acceptance, approval and love, attempting to cope through anorexia nervosa is hardly surprising.

''My parents are real . . . expecting of perfection,'' says Alison. ''There were always a lot of pretty high expectations in my family, that whatever you did, whatever you were interested in, you had to be the *best*. My mother has her own business, and it was always like I had to be a miniature version of my mother. My family was kind of like a monarchy, because my mom was *the* controller, and she told my father what to tell me, so it was like having a duplicate of my mother in my father.''

As Alison describes, a young girl growing up in an achievement-oriented household perceives her parents—and thus, the world—to be conditional in their acceptance, approval, and love for her, she copes the only way she knows how. She creates a ''false self,'' a mask to wear, to play a part that she believes will please her parents and significant others. In other words, she becomes whatever she thinks ''they'' want her to be.

''Whatever I did, it was always for my parents,'' Alison explains. ''I was a real people-pleaser growing up. I wanted to be the best in the class, so the teacher would like me, so I would get good grades and my parents would be proud of me.''

Unfortunately, the false self that Alison created, like that of all anorexics, is merely a shell. It's her mask, her disguise, as she acts her role and plays her part to earn the respect, acknowledgment, approval, and love she so desperately craves.

When the anorexic woman doesn't get the response she's after, she strives to make the shell even more perfect. But this role, this life she is leading is not her own. There's no tolerance for flaws, for mistakes, for failures. Like an actress, she cannot break character, she cannot dare let down her guard to reveal her true impulses and feelings. Being "real," being "authentic," are alien concepts.

The most unfortunate consequence is that the love the anorexic craves more than anything can never be felt, can never get through to her because the mask, the false self, is being praised and acknowledged. As she hides behind the mask of her false self, she cannot develop self-esteem, a cohesive identity, or a sense of self-worth, because as researcher W. Nicholson Browning (1985) points out, her false self is being accepted and acknowledged, while her true self is hidden from view.[1]

Nothing the anorexic woman does is initiated because *she* wants it. Rather, it's motivated largely by the desire to please other people, to make them happy and proud, to earn their acceptance, approval, and love. That is why she fails to develop a healthy sense of her own identity, her strengths and weaknesses, or who she really is. The woman the anorexic has become has been largely determined by the expectations she has perceived in others.

For Robin, the false self came into play at mealtimes. "My mother comes from a family that believes people should eat lots of food," Robin explains, "so she would always prepare large amounts of food. But there was always a feeling that I had there at home, for some reason, that it was not okay to go back for seconds and to eat a normal-sized meal. That just came from comments that my mother would make — maybe at my brothers — to imply that they were being greedy or something if they ate a large portion. And so somehow, I just developed a fear of eating in front of her."

"When I'd go out places, I'd eat food a lot, so then when I would go home at mealtimes, I would only eat small amounts of food," Robin says. "Then my mother would not have anything to say. It didn't feel like it at that time, but I was trying to please my mother in some way."

As an anorexic's false self strives to please and secure the love and approval of her father, mother, and significant others, her true impulses, her true self remain submerged. Her genuine urges of self-assertion—of standing up to others who are overstepping boundaries—are stifled. She develops a habit of acquiescing to others' demands because the alternative is terrifying. If she disagrees or stands up to others, she fears she'll lose their love.

In Heidi's case, it was too threatening to express true feelings, to be in conflict in her family, so she kept her mouth shut. "At home, my mom is in charge," says Heidi. "There's no question whatsoever. It's a very traditional split-up—my father is the breadwinner and my mother is the housewife. And you know, Dad takes orders from her at home. I didn't perceive my mother to be tyrannically controlling, but I could never really stand up to her and say 'no.' I couldn't stand up to her in an argument ever. I still can't."

However, it's not that the mothers of anorexics are overly controlling, manipulative, possessive, cruel, ruthless, erratic, and unable to properly "mirror" their daughters—a portrait that popular "ego psychological" theorists maintain. Rather, I believe the familial factor that makes a young girl vulnerable to anorexia nervosa centers more on conditional love. The daughter grows up convinced that she must meet absolute standards of perfection to *earn* the love and approval of significant others. Consequently, her behavior, her drive and ambition hinges on whatever is necessary to please others, not her own needs and desires.

"Family systems" theorists miss the point as well, by making broad, sweeping generalizations that all "anorexic families" are highly enmeshed, superficially nice and harmonious, extremely rigid and overprotective. Some, maybe. But certainly not all.

"I come from an abusive home," Chiara explains, "and I thought that if I was the good girl, did well in school, was perfect, then maybe I wouldn't get hurt. It was also a rebellion against what they said about me, because my mother would say I'd turn out just like my dad, who's no good, and my mother's relatives and family would say the same thing . . . because I looked like him, I acted like him. So I had to prove them wrong. I had to refute everything they said about me. I was always trying to overcome their predictions. I wasn't going to let them be right. All those achievements and accomplishments were to prove that they were wrong.''

School became a haven for Chiara. Because she didn't hear praise, acknowledgment, or encouragement at home, she turned to her teachers at school for it, and was motivated to earn their acceptance and approval. ''When I wanted to go to college, my mother said, 'Why are you going to go to college? You're just going to get married and get pregnant and have kids. Then what are you going to do with that degree? What good is it?' So I never got any encouragement. I never heard, 'Wow, this is a great report card!' or 'You're really doing well!' I never had any kind of measuring stick at home as to what was good and what was bad. I just knew that if I did well, that would give me a better chance of getting out.''

After Chiara's sexually abusive, alcoholic father deserted the family, her mother went on public assistance and Chiara stopped eating. ''I felt lonely and misunderstood—the scapegoat,'' she says. ''I think I was the scapegoat of the family because I reminded my mother so much of my dad and she never really resolved any of those issues with him. Or she felt so hurt that she put it all back on me.''

In other ''atypical'' family situations, the women I talked with felt the most accurate description of their family life was having parents who were ''not really there'' for them—physically or emotionally.

Jenny resented that her mother wasn't always available. ''My mother was never there for anything,'' she says bitterly. ''She was always working. My mom worked on weekends and she was always, always working. I don't take that out on her—she's gone a long way, and she still does a lot of work, and you know, we needed the money. But she just never . . . she wasn't even caring. She wouldn't even come home and make me dinner. 'Oh, make a Lean Cuisine, honey.' I was like, 'What is this attitude? You're my mother; I'm supposed to be eating nutritious food.' But it was just, we were second and work was first. So I felt kind of ignored.

''And I didn't take it out on her,'' Jenny stresses, ''I'm not angry with her now or anything like that. She was always buying us clothes and stuff like that, but it's just, the attention was given through clothes and money, and not her.

"I just didn't feel I was getting any attention, and I think that's where it all started," she finally concludes. "I just felt I needed something to *prove* that I was there."

Many women, like Jenny, did *not* grow up in a *Leave It to Beaver* household with a stay-at-home mom. Yet one must resist the urge to pin the blame on the "working mom." The real issue is whether a child feels emotional support from one or both parents — a variable which operates quite independently of a mother's or father's employment status.

Given the widely varying family backgrounds these women describe, it is clear that neither the "ego-psychological" nor "family systems" theories of anorexia nervosa hold up in all cases. In fact, with the spiraling number of reported cases of anorexia nervosa over the last twenty years, researchers Donald W. Schwartz, Michael G. Thompson, and Craig L. Johnson (1982) contend that citing "ego-psychological" or "family systems" theories to explain this dramatic increase is absurd, as it implies that over the last two decades, we have, for some reason, seen either an epidemic of erratic and unempathetic mothers or highly enmeshed, overprotective families.[2]

Granted, the illogic implicit in either of these premises *does* seem ridiculous. Factors within the family are but one piece of the very complex puzzle of anorexia nervosa; they are not the entire puzzle. Families alone cannot explain why one becomes anorexic.

Yet the proclivity toward creating a false self and coping through an addictive strategy such as anorexia nervosa, *is* bred in a particular type of family environment — one, I believe, that the daughter perceives as extremely conditional, in which she must *earn* love and approval. The important point is that regardless of what her parents actually intended or how unconditional they truly felt in their love, the daughter perceives it as conditional. This, in combination with her very low self-esteem and relentless perfectionism, leads her to behave in ways that do not reflect her own needs and desires, but rather, with whatever she believes will please others and earn her acceptance, approval, and love.

"I'd think that I'd make them happy if I did something just right," explains Alison, "but it always seemed like whenever I got to that point where I thought I had everything under control and that I'd get their constant approval, it seemed like even *that* wasn't enough."

Perfection, of course, is impossible to achieve, and comparing herself to these absolute standards only lowers a woman's self-esteem even more. She feels horrible about herself—that she's a worthless, disappointing failure. Yet she remains firm in her convictions that the way to secure unconditional love and approval—once and for all—is to be absolutely, totally perfect.

The conditions a woman believes she must attain in order to earn the acceptance, approval, and love she wants more than anything only escalate. She has to be better—more perfect—and then she will be loved. But it's never enough. A woman's externally-directed behavior patterns are magnified when she turns to anorexia nervosa as a coping strategy.

Chapter 4

Onset

Chiara was only ten when she began dieting. "I'd have note-books and calorie counters hidden in the pantry—ten years old!" she exclaims, "and I'd have to go back there after every meal and write down everything and it couldn't go over a certain number of calories. Somehow, I thought, 'This is somewhere where I can get control.'"

Chiara, like nearly one out of five women in the U.S., was sexu-ally abused by a family member as a child.[1] "I remember strange things with eating when I was ten," she says, "but it was also around that age that the physical and sexual abuse started to get bad. I was so hurt by it—this is only looking back on it now—that I blocked it out of my mind completely.

"I wanted control someplace," Chiara adds reflectively. "It was like if I got thin enough, then maybe nobody would notice me and I wouldn't get hurt. I got so frightened when I started to go into puberty, because then I would get a woman's body. That was an-other big part of it—going into puberty around 12 years old and then men starting to notice me. And I thought, 'Well, if they do what my dad does to me, maybe I have to stop it and get really thin.'"

From the time she was a little girl, Alison had been tormented by taunts and criticism about her weight. "I had been taking dance, pretty much since I was three or four," she says, "and I got a lot of comments and things like that from my dance instructor and got really pushed into losing weight. And a lot of other people were telling me that if I were thinner, I'd be more flexible, if I were thinner, I'd be a better dancer. Most of it was criticism, I guess."

In the beginning, losing weight was something Alison had to

work hard at. "I was pretty sensible about it, just dieting and eating lots of salads. I got a lot of encouragement from my dance instructor and the other girls in my dance class, because the more weight I lost, the better I was at dancing. I was more flexible, and things like that.

"At the beginning, I could see the weight loss, because it was pretty dramatic," Alison adds. "But as I got closer, I always felt I needed to lose a little more. I'd set a limit, and when I got there, I wasn't happy, so I'd set another one. And when other dancers would tell me they were jealous of me because I was thin, I didn't see how possibly, because I thought I was so fat. I didn't think of myself as being thin, because I wasn't thin *enough*. I was pretty overweight — about 190 — and then I lost . . . down to 72."

Heidi began losing weight after she lost her best friend to another girl. "I had a very good friend, my best friend. She went to my church but to another junior high," she explains. "Then we had another friend who went to our church, and who went to my best friend's junior high also. It used to be the two of us, then it was the three of us, and then it sort of shifted around to the two of *them*.

"One thing the three of us were always trying to do was diet," Heidi says. "When the two of them started going away, it was the same time I got my braces and my headgear and I *couldn't* eat, and I was dropping weight like crazy. I was 14 . . . 15. And that's how I felt I won out on them. It just started that way . . . and it kept going. I dropped 50 pounds — down to 75 — in nine months."

Jenny says she was trying to get a little attention when she began dieting. "My sister was going through this really awful period where she was turning into a delinquent. She was really rebellious, dying her hair, going out with her friends, skipping school, and all that kind of stuff," Jenny recalls. "Also, a close relative was really ill that year and she died. So my parents were really wrapped up in that, and wrapped up with my sister and trying to control her. Her teachers were calling every night and saying, 'Your daughter was not in class today,' and they were really wrapped up in her. And that's when I felt I wasn't getting any attention."

At first, Jenny tried to be the *opposite* of her sister — the perfect little angel, "the best little girl in the world." "There I was, this perfect child," she remarks. "I'd come home and make dinner every night."

But "the best little girl" routine didn't work. It wasn't enough to get the response she was after. "I got obsessed in the kitchen. I was making stuff for other people and shoving it on them. I just didn't feel I was getting any attention," she says, "and I think that's where it all started."

A geographical move triggered Yvette's initial weight loss. "When I was 15, we moved from a large city to a very rural area," Yvette recalls. "It was a major move and a wrenching experience, because I was *in* school and we were more or less settled down, and I had to start all over again in — pardon my bluntness — a very lower-class area. It was not as stimulating or as challenging in terms of the quality of the school or the people.

"I felt like an outsider, almost like an invader," Yvette adds. "And definitely not wanted, because we moved to a small community and people were very chilly to newcomers. It was a difficult experience trying to be accepted and coping with that whole feeling of being rejected. When I was 15 — that's when we moved — I remember I just stopped eating. I don't think I ate for a month. I got *really* skinny."

Jill was confused and uncertain about her future after dropping out of college. "I spent two years there, not being really sure of what I wanted to do in college or what I was taking these classes for," she says. "So I dropped out and I had a couple of bad relationships."

After experiencing two devastating break-ups, there was no place for the hurt to manifest itself. "I didn't know how to express the pain that I felt from being rejected and didn't understand why the relationship was severed because it was their decision that it would be severed," Jill says. "In one relationship, I saw him with another woman. He wasn't physically doing anything with her, but the fact that he was lying to me hurt me so much that I wanted to die. I felt lied to and didn't know how to express it. At that time, I was really into yoga and vegetarianism and things like that. And that's when I really got into fasting."

Robin was going through a great deal of emotional turmoil after finishing college. "I had just graduated from college and I was having a hard time finding a full-time job," she remembers. "Also, I had just moved into an apartment with someone I had been dating throughout college and that relationship was having a lot of problems. And at the same time, I was trying to relocate. I was under a lot of pressure trying to find somewhere else to move. There was a lot of stress going on, and it seemed food was the one thing I could be in control of," Robin says. "I felt I did not need anybody else and I could not trust anybody else. *I* was the only person I could trust, so I just built my own little world around myself. I was actually destroying myself, but it didn't seem that way at the time."

Chelsey had experienced several emotional losses and other stresses in her life. "They weren't big losses really, just people moving away that I was close to—two people at the same time," she says. "Then I had been married about nine months at the time, and I guess I was having the usual early marriage kinds of problems. I was feeling inadequate at work around the same time, and it was sort of everything all at once."

Chelsey says dieting was a conscious undertaking to try to feel better about herself. "I'd always wanted to be really thin, ever since I was little," she explains. "I'd always admired women that were really skinny. And I was just kind of depressed and lonely and needed something to focus on and make myself feel good, and that's what it was.

"I just thought . . . I wanted to lose weight," Chelsey says. "I was getting disgusted—I'd gained three pounds at that time, which on a short person shows. It seemed like I was a few pounds over, and I thought, 'Well, if I lose five pounds, I'll be *perfect.*' So I just put all of my efforts into losing weight and it was real easy, you know, a lot easier than I thought. And then I didn't want to stop."

Leslie began restricting her food intake soon after she was raped. "That's when I can see it *really* started getting bad," she remembers. "I just started getting this fear of fat, like, 'God, I don't want to be fat!' I told myself, 'No, you're not hungry. If you eat, you're going to get so *fat*, and you're going to have to exercise more, so you might as well not eat it.' I *denied* being hungry. And I began exercising even more. I reached a point where I was exercising five times a day. It was just a feeling of, 'Oh God, I don't want to be this fat, I need to lose weight!'"

Leslie blamed herself for the rape, which isn't surprising, considering our societal conditioning. As Linda Tschirhart Sanford and Mary Ellen Donovan point out in *Women & Self-Esteem*, the American criminal justice system has traditionally put the victim on trial, rather than the rapist. This, in turn, leads the woman (and public-at-large) to conclude that *she* is at fault, that she was in the "wrong place at the wrong time," that she was "asking for it."[2]

"I was feeling . . . just *guilty*," says Leslie, "like I must have done something to provoke it . . . that I was *bad*. And I was just married. I thought, 'Oh gosh, you've ruined your marriage.' I didn't tell anybody, for almost a year."

The shame kept Leslie quiet. She was afraid to tell anyone. So she tried to hide her secret, to hush it and suppress it from surfacing. And in the beginning, she was quite successful: no one sensed anything was wrong. To her friends and family, Leslie was dieting—and everyone was applauding. "When you start losing weight, people really reinforce it," Leslie remarks. "They say, 'Oh, you lost weight—you look really good.' I'd think, 'Oh yeah!' And it just kept me going."

But it wasn't just dieting. Leslie was shrinking herself, trying to become smaller, more invisible, so that men wouldn't notice her and she wouldn't be victimized again. "If I focused on food and eating, then I wouldn't have to focus on any other issues that were really going on that I needed to address," she remarks. "It was a way that I could block everything out. Because I was so wrapped up in food . . . and once that kicked in, it was an easy way for me to not have to think about things."

Nancy, who became anorexic at age 40, was experiencing a lot of tension on the job and in her personal life. "Things started happening at work and I was having problems there. I got transferred in my job and at the time, it felt like a demotion to me, and so that was bothering me," Nancy says. "And a friend of mine became seriously ill and he died. Then my husband became seriously ill and at the same time, they told me I was going to have to take a demotion at work, so all of this hit me all at once. That was when the weight loss really accelerated. I thought this was one thing that I could control."

As the above stories indicate, anorexia nervosa is a desperate attempt at control . . . when everything else seems to be caving in, slipping away, and falling apart. Regardless of each woman's stage in life or the personal life stress that triggers her bout with anorexia, all speak in the same voice because the aftermath is always the same.

Feeling extremely fragile and vulnerable, overwhelmed by pressure, anxiety, and confusion, these women experience the merciless effects of life's ravaging blows, of being knocked down one time too many. That's why controlling weight is so appealing, so alluring at this time in their lives. When everything seems so uncertain, so confusing, so out-of-control, this sense of control is something these women can count on, that will make them feel better, that will always be there and will never let them down.

Women have enough going against them in society. Magazines and other media constantly tell women that they're not pretty enough, not glamorous enough, not thin enough. The corporate world still pays women, on average, a scant two-thirds of what men make. Contemporary cultural mandates call on women to be "Superwomen," to do everything perfectly, to work a double-day, performing the bulk of the housework in addition to holding full-time jobs.

With all of these pressures, it's hard to continually react like a Romper Room punching-bag clown — to get punched and bounce back, get punched and bounce back, get punched and bounce back. Sometimes those blows knock the wind right out of a woman. Sometimes they stab and puncture a woman until there's no air left, and that's when she's vulnerable to anorexia nervosa. When women don't have the strength or resources to get themselves off the ropes while they're being "beaten up" from all sides they resort to whatever strategy they can think of to regain some feeling of control in their lives. For women who become anorexic, the coping mechanism is controlling their weight.

Part of the appeal of losing weight is that it's a sure thing. It is mathematical—a fact of modern science—that if you take in less calories than you expend, you lose weight. It is that simple, that controllable, that certain. Plus, it is one thing that the anorexic can feel completely in charge of—many for the first time. Many feel great power in knowing that they alone decide how much or how little to eat in a day. When the needle on the scale goes down, the anorexic is responsible for the weight loss. No one else can take credit for it.

"It was like, I did it myself, I think," remarks Deborah, "I just liked watching the scale go down, I liked watching the numbers go down. I felt that I'd achieved something every day."

It's something a woman can feel completely in charge of, for once. "Losing weight was one thing that *I* could control," Nancy remarks. "I could stand on the scale and say, 'Okay, this is what I weigh today; tomorrow I can weigh half a pound less, or even a whole pound less, if I don't eat.'"

Invariably, the process always starts out the same. "I was just going to lose a little weight in the beginning," Nikki recalls. "I just wanted to lose five pounds or so. Then I thought I'd be perfect. But I lost ten pounds. And then I got under 100. And then I wanted to see what it was like to be in the lower half of the 90s, and then in the 80s, until I was keeping track of everything I ate every day, what I weighed every day, how many calories I'd eaten, and how much I'd exercised."

Losing weight hooks the anorexic. If a woman has never done anything for herself, if she has always strived to please other people, to be whatever she thought "they" wanted her to be, it's the first time she does something because she wanted it, no one else. The ensuing success is positively exhilarating. She feels so elated, so in charge, that she wants to keep on doing it because it makes her feel good about herself, and her life. Dieting makes the anorexic feel special. Losing weight is "her thing," her identity, and she doesn't want anyone else doing it, as Nancy illustrates.

"One night, my friend and I had gone out to dinner," Nancy

remembers. "She was in from a trip and I had picked her up at the airport. A couple of nights later, we went out to dinner together, and she made some comment about losing weight—that she herself needed to lose weight. And the thought went through my mind, 'She can't do that, that's my thing! That's my special thing!' And then all of a sudden, even when I was thinking that, I thought, 'That's funny, why should I think that?' And I looked at what she was eating—a perfectly regular meal—steak, baked potato, sour cream and all of that—and I was having a salad. And then I thought, 'Hmmm. Maybe there's something not quite right here. I *have* been eating a lot of salad. But I wanted to lose weight, and I've been doing okay with it.' So I wasn't worried."

Anorexics get caught up in denial, like any other addict. All an anorexic wants is to feel better about herself, to *like* herself, to be happy. As Hilde Bruch (1973) notes, since she feels that "being too fat" is the root of all her problems, the cause of her despair, she tries desperately to correct this flaw. But no matter how much weight she loses, it is never enough to give her the inner reassurance, self-esteem and acceptance she wants so desperately. So the downward spiral continues.[3]

"I wanted to be thin," remarks Helena. "I started just to eat less and less. And then I wanted to be 'the best one' who didn't eat. I was an au pair in Switzerland—I cared for a little boy of two years and I thought I had to eat less than he. So I did."

When the obsession takes over, the anorexic has to be *the best* at losing weight. She twists things in her head so that hunger is *satisfying*, because it's clear evidence of her continuing achievement. The gnawing hunger pangs actually encourage her to go on, luring her with the possibility that tomorrow, the scale will go even lower.

"I would be starving—*starving*!" Jenny admits. "I'd have headaches all the time and my eyes would be bulging out of my head. But the hunger made me feel *good*. I thought, 'I'm doing something; I'm losing weight.' In my head, I turned it into such a satisfying feeling, to have my stomach growling, and I would just ignore it and do something else instead of eat. And people would say, 'How can you do that?' Well it's easy if you're determined to do that. You can *easily* ignore it."

Watching the numbers go down on the scale every day is the high that the anorexic is on. It's what she lives for, the only thing in her life that means anything. The discipline of this acute self-denial makes the anorexic feel *good*. Some women feel proud and special and *superior*, because they are successfully losing weight — something that no one can seem to achieve as well.

"I'd even feel superior in the grocery store," Robin laughs. "All I'd have in my cart were vegetables and fruits, and I'd see all these people with pies and sodas. I'd feel proud and superior whenever people would make comments to me about being underweight. *That* was such a compliment to me. Being thin."

After a while, anorexic women feel positively omnipotent. "Most of the women at work were overweight," remarks Nancy, "and I remember going in there and beginning to feel very superior to them. I thought, 'Ha! You're all so fat! No wonder! Look at what you're eating! See, all I'm having is salad and I'm going to be much better off this way.' So I kept losing and losing weight."

Eventually other people keep getting in the way, trying to interfere with an anorexic's special achievement. "People started making comments, 'Gee, you're getting awfully thin,' 'You're not eating much — is that all you're going to eat?'" Nancy remembers. "My husband really didn't notice too much because he was working two jobs and I was working two jobs, so that we came and went kind of like this [missing each other]. When we *did* eat together, it was usually on the weekends, and usually, I would eat normally in front of him, or what he perceived as normal. By that time, it was getting to be colder weather, so I was wearing layers and sweaters and stuff, and he couldn't see how thin I was. He didn't realize anything was going on."

Nancy was successful in camouflaging her secret. "Then along about December, I started reading books," she says. "I started looking up anorexia. Well, of course I thought I *couldn't* be anorexic. At that point, I was 40 years old. I thought, 'I'm 40 years old and I haven't lost 25 percent of my body weight, and I haven't lost my period.'" Although Nancy did not yet meet the clinical definition of anorexia nervosa, her behavior was clearly leading her down that path. At this stage, the anorexic starts playing games with herself. *She* doesn't have to adhere to the laws of science.

They apply to *average* people — the common masses — and she is not average.

Nancy was just . . . well, different. She read in nutritional textbooks and medical journals that a human being could not subsist on a certain number of calories. Nancy thought, " 'Now what do *they* know? They've never done it! I'm doing fine. I'm doing fine on two or three hundred calories.' I always felt like, 'They don't really *know*!' "

As the anorexic reaches her goal weight, she distorts her body image so that she can keep losing weight and keep feeling a fleeting sense of esteem. When the anorexic examines herself in the mirror, she does not see emaciation, but only "fat zones" — hips and thighs and buttocks that she *has* to lose so she can continue to achieve — doing the one thing in her life that no one else is in charge of, that no one can control.

"My main attention always went to my thighs," says Robin. "I would not be thin enough until I lost all of my thighs. And no matter how much weight I lost, I could not get rid of them. That's how I saw it. It all just kind of went around that."

Nancy says it was never *that* bad for her. "I never really had . . . well, I don't like my stomach sticking out, but I never . . . well, my rear end, I don't like my rear end to be too big, but I never did get overly focused like some women who don't like their thighs being too big or whatever," she says. "It was just that the thinner I got, the more I enjoyed seeing my thighs getting thinner and my stomach getting flatter and concave and all of that. It was a sign that I was getting thin — nice and thin."

The obsession with being "nice and thin" took Nancy over completely. "I used to sit at my desk and think, 'Let's see, I had orange juice and I had coffee, and that's going to be a hundred calories,' " Nancy recalls. " 'Then if I have such and such for lunch, and such and such . . . well, maybe I'd better not have lunch. Or if I *do* have lunch, maybe I'd better skip having the whatever.' I was so full of all these thoughts — and I'm the world's worst mathematician. I *hate* math, and here I am, calculating all this stuff. And then a customer would come and ask me something and I couldn't care less what the customer wanted. I was too busy trying to figure out if

I should eat 200 calories for lunch or 100. I can remember sitting there thinking, 'Wow, I'm 79, I wonder if I can get to 78? I wonder what would happen if I got to 75?'"

What starts as a simple coping strategy quickly becomes an obsession, filling the void in an anorexic's life and becoming the center of her existence.

"At my worst, my day would start off with a cup of coffee, and I would drink half of that cup of coffee," Robin remembers. "Back at that time, I would put a dash of creamer in it — just one little dash. And I would have a piece of fruit — let's say one orange. I would section off the orange and that orange would last me for two or three days. So for breakfast, I might have two sections of one full orange, something like that. And pretty much, that's all I would have during the morning time.

"And lunchtime, I might eat soup," Robin recounts. "It would be Campbell's soup — it would always be tomato — with a lot of water in it. I'd measure it out and have no more than six ounces total soup. I'd have one saltless saltine cracker with that. During the day, I might have another half a cup of coffee. For a while, I would drink chicken broth — have like part of a cup of that.

"For dinner, I would fix a very tiny salad, just with lettuce, a little bit of tomato, just a couple of things," Robin remembers. "Again, I would have soup — six ounces of soup — one cracker, and if I had meat, it would be less than an ounce of meat. My main calories came during the later evening time. I couldn't let myself eat any more from that time, up until 11 o'clock. And at that time, I would eat maybe a half a donut or a couple of cookies, something like that.

"During my most severe time of restricting, I would exercise *a lot*," Robin recalls. "I got to the point where I would have to exercise before I could allow myself to eat one of those meals, just to take a coffee break. Coffee and a little bit of fruit. After I would have that, I would have to exercise again. I would just exercise there in the apartment, maybe for about a half an hour, just stretches and things like that.

"The nights at 11 o'clock when I would have a half a donut or something," Robin adds, "maybe a few times, I would have a *whole* donut, and to me, I had really binged. That was a binge to me. I'd feel really guilty and I'd likely exercise more. The next day, I would eat less to make up for it."

By focusing so much on food, weight and thinness, Robin could forget all the pain, confusion, and anger. She could focus all of her attention, all of her energy on losing weight and block everything else completely out of her mind.

"With my eating disorder, I numbed myself to all my feelings and just totally denied that I could possibly have any feelings," Robin remarks. "I didn't want to feel anything because I thought it would all be painful for some reason. I was trying to protect myself from this unknown pain."

Consequently, as Robin's weight plummeted lower and lower, she became increasingly isolated. She couldn't eat in front of other people, because she felt others were watching her and commenting on how little she ate. "As I restricted more and more, I interacted less and less with people," Robin recalls, "so that people wouldn't . . . well, I was afraid that if I socialized with people, that would encourage me to eat more because that's what I saw. It seemed like people would get together and they would like to go out and eat and drink and things like that. So I just avoided those situations."

When anorexia nervosa takes over, losing weight is the only thing that matters, the only thing that exists in an anorexic's world. She clings to it desperately, because her thinness defines her, it differentiates her from others. It's her identity and all she really has. Without that, there is nothing . . . nothing that means anything to her.

There's no room for anything or anyone else. "I just didn't want to deal with people," Heidi remarks. "I could run for miles and miles, but I can remember that smiling was such an exhausting thing to me. I couldn't smile, much less keep up a conversation with anybody. I just didn't want to be bothered with anyone.

"I was so depressed all the time — the word I would use is

'gray,'" Heidi says. "Every morning I would wake up and everything was gray, no matter what. Losing weight was something I felt driven to do, but I didn't really want anybody's attention while I was doing it. I just wanted to be left alone. What I really wanted was just to fade away. I remember thinking that . . . wishing I could just fade away. I would not consider suicide — I couldn't do that: I just wanted to fade away and not exist."

Chapter 5

Chronicity

When anorexia nervosa becomes intrinsically tied to a woman's identity, she clings to it desperately—because it's all she feels she has. "I felt this is my thing, this is my life," says Helena. "I equaled anorexia. That was my identity." That's *precisely* why anorexia nervosa is so difficult to overcome. Anorexic women define themselves through it.

"Anorexia is *doing* something," Monica remarks. "It's very concrete. You lose weight, you see results. For me—this is really sick—it's like winning the Nobel Prize or something. It's like you get a kingdom or become a goddess. I felt that way because I felt I was so bad, I couldn't do anything right. The only thing I could do right was starving maybe. I felt it was to *be* someone, like I was becoming a unique person, creating my own identity. You feel that you are nobody before, and when you starve, you're getting yourself down to the bones: 'This is really me. This is really what I am.'"

Some women feel that anorexia is their identity. "I don't personally feel I'm trying my absolute hardest in getting over this, because I still want to hang onto it," remarks Jenny. "It's my toy, it's my game, it's *mine*! And I'm not going to give it up. The one thing with exercise is that no one can take it away from me. I can do that every single day for four hours and nobody can come out to my apartment and chain me down, strap me to my bed and say, 'You are *not* going walking today.' They can't do it. They cannot do it. That is *mine*. That's all *mine*. And that makes me feel wonderful!"

Jenny admits she *could* recover if she wanted to. "I do admit that I'm not working as hard as I could," she says. "If I sat down every day and wrote down all my thoughts and really sat here and worked on it, maybe it would go a lot faster. But then when I get into school, I've got a hundred other things on my mind, and they all come first. Food goes to the back of my mind. That is the last thing on my mind, you know? I'll deal with that later. This is more important. These grades are more important. This class is more important. This date is more important. The food can wait. The food can wait. The food can wait.''

In addition to feeling in control, another reason for putting off recovery is apparent in Jenny's voice. As she continues to starve herself and persevere in her personal hunger strike, Jenny can drive her parents crazy. She can make them pay for the lack of attention she perceived.

"Here I am, just giving my parents another $70 bill," Jenny says, almost gleefully. "Every week. Another psychiatrist and another month of pills. I feel *a little* guilty about that," Jenny admits. "Because I know I'm not pushing myself as much as I could. I know that. Because I still want to hang on to this."

Obviously, Jenny is getting something out of it. She stays anorexic because she believes the payoffs are worth far more than stopping it. For some anorexics, as in Jenny's case, it could be the need to gain attention; a desperate plea to get someone to notice her. For others the payoff comes from differentiating themselves as human beings—carving their own niches, and finding their own unique identity. This is very important to many women, taught to piggyback their identities on others—as in "So-and-So's daughter," "So-and-So's girlfriend," and "So-and-So's wife." By becoming an anorexic, a woman is striving to accomplish something completely on her own.

The "payoffs" vary among women. Some anorexics feel more attractive by attempting to meet sociocultural mandates of extreme thinness as a standard of beauty. Or perhaps, like Monica, they are starving themselves in order to be nurtured and taken care of. "When I was little, my parents were very concerned about their marriage," says Monica, "and I had to be the strong one to take care of their feelings and to comfort them. I think I lost some years in my childhood, so I wanted to be small, I wanted to be little so people would take care of me, hug me, and treat me like a baby almost."

Jill identifies with this theme as well. "The only part of thinness that I enjoyed was that I was then able to feel that I was vulnerable," Jill remarks. "I could make mistakes. I wasn't totally responsible. The weight bought me an excuse. It wasn't something where I felt I would be more accepted if I were that thin. It was that I would *not* be accepted. I *would* need to be taken care of. Someone would say, 'I'll take care of you, I'll give you more time to get your life together. You aren't capable of taking care of yourself, so I'll take care of you.'"

Other anorexic women, however, try to take care of *themselves*, by seeking protection in a hostile environment. This is a recurrent theme among survivors of sexual abuse, who were *not* trying to attract attention, but to shrink away from it—most particularly, from *male* attention. "I wanted to be so thin that people wouldn't notice me," Leslie remarks, "so that *men* wouldn't notice me." Leslie believed that by getting smaller and taking up less space, she would become invisible, and maybe—just maybe—she wouldn't get hurt again.

The underlying messages a woman may be trying to convey through anorexia nervosa are very diverse. They cannot be pigeonholed into neat little categories of *always* being this, or *always* being that, as many clinicians maintain. The underlying meaning depends on the individual woman. Yet a common theme emerges through their voices: all have adopted a coping strategy to survive in a world that is hostile to women—that limits their opportunities, that teaches them to define themselves through appearance, and through other people. At a time when it all seems too much, when everything feels so precarious, uncertain, and out-of-control, anorexia nervosa seems to offer the perfect escape.

"When I became anorexic, I felt pushed into a corner. I felt [a great deal of] pressure and I felt I had to hide," Monica remarks. "I had some unconscious thought that I had to really make myself sick—so that all the demands that people wanted from me, they couldn't have, because they would see that I am sick. So I'd get some kind of holiday from life. And if you have lots of anxiety, bad feelings and everything, it's perfect to be anorexic, because then you have no time to think or to feel. You just get so banged up, you can't think about anything. All your time goes to not eating and exercising.''

For once in her life, an anorexic woman feels she has control, because she is controlling everything in regard to her food intake — how much or how little she will eat. "Anorexic behavior means control,'' says Chiara. "I have control. It's thinking that I can control my food and control my body. When everything else feels out of control, this is the one thing I really can control.''

Anorexia nervosa becomes Chiara's fortress, her armor. "It's like I get so numb and shut myself off to those feelings so that no one can hurt me," says Chiara. "It's almost like I get so frightened that someone is going to hurt me, that I have to shut it off so no one can. It's like I've become invisible.'' No one can get through to Chiara. Nothing can reach her, nothing can hurt her, nothing can stop her.

Forced intervention attempts are futile at this point, because the anorexic woman is caught up in denial. Relentlessly pursuing the ultimate state of thinness makes her world go round. It gives her life meaning and she'll do whatever it takes to hold onto her anorexia. Getting carted off to therapists or thrown into hospitals only provokes her intense fighting spirit. How *dare* anyone try to rob her of the only thing she feels she's got!

Chronic anorexics like Annett become cynical and obstinate and delight in outsmarting therapists and the medical establishment. "I go to psychologists and just tell them what they want to hear,'' laughs Annett. "I've read a certain amount of psychology texts, so I know what I'm supposed to say and how I'm supposed to react. What they want to hear is that I am doing so well and managing everything. So I tell them I'm doing things I'm really not doing, just to make them happy. I tell them it's been 'very, very hard work,' but I've been doing it. It's very good theatre. You get very good at lying.''

Besides lying, another popular stance among anorexics is refusing to say anything at all to therapists. "I was *the* angry bitch,'' says Alison. "I was so mad at my parents for taking me to a psychologist that I refused to answer any questions, so I didn't. Until *I* decided that I needed to see a therapist, I was totally resistant to anything and everything. I totally denied that I had any sort of a problem." With denial, of course, comes deception. And anorexics — like all addicts — are particularly adept at coming up with all sorts of innovative schemes to "pull one over" on the medical profession.

Nancy was warned repeatedly by her doctor that if she went below 85 pounds, she'd land herself in the hospital for the third time around. "I was *not* going to do that again," she says adamantly. "Summer was coming and I was *not* going to spend it in the hospital. So I started playing a few tricks. I bought these weights that you tie into your running shoes — you put them in your laces. I took one apart and discovered that it was a neat little package — about a half a pound of weight," Nancy explains. "The first week, I was a little bit under, but I knew that the nutritionist weighed me fully clothed, so I thought, 'No problem.' I went in with an extra pound taped into my underwear."

The following week, Nancy lost *more* weight, so she simply taped in another pound of weights. This went on all summer and it could have gone on indefinitely, but in September, another anorexic who knew Nancy's secret called the doctor and turned her in. (Her friend said she was "worried," but Nancy suspected she was just a little jealous.)

"At the end, I was waddling in to my nutritionist weighing, she thought, around 89 or 90," Nancy says with a grin. "In fact, I weighed around 77 or 78. See, the nutritionist was new and not experienced with anorexics. She didn't know you're going to do this kind of thing when you're desperate."

After a while, nothing seems taboo or off-limits. As the case of Linda illustrates, the desperation to lose weight intensifies. It gets harder and harder to lose weight, and anorexics sometimes turn to abusing laxatives, diuretics, and over-the-counter diet pills.

"I used to go into supermarkets late at night and slip packages of Dexatrim into my purse," Linda admits. "I was going to school at the time and didn't have enough money to buy them. Plus, I felt a little embarrassed *buying* them, because the check-out clerks always looked at me kind of strangely. I'd go to a different supermarket every night and pocket laxatives and diuretics and diet pills — sometimes hitting several different stores in one night. I liked

NoDoze, too, because they kept me awake late at night when I was really exhausted and needed to study.''

Other anorexics just as desperate as Linda, sometimes resort to syrup of Ipecac, a potentially lethal poison remedy, or sticking their fingers down their throats, just to make sure that whatever was eaten in a binge, won't show up on the scale the next morning. (This kind of purging differs from that of bulimics, who consume enormous amounts of food and then vomit. Anorexics may purge any little bit of food that they perceive to be a "binge" — a regular meal, or one cracker too many.)

"One time, we went out for dinner," Joanna recalls, "and everything was fine until my husband insisted I have dessert. So I ate dessert, and when we got home, I told him I was going to take a walk. I went out for a nice long walk, and then found a place and made myself vomit. Another time, I used Ipecac. That was nasty. Nasty! So I only did that once."

Anorexics are caught up in denial when they begin practicing such behaviors. An anorexic woman may hear the words "anorexia nervosa," but she doesn't have it. Not her. Not *that* bad.

"My doctor wanted me to be hospitalized," says Chelsey. "That was his recommendation, but I just sort of refused because I didn't think it was necessary. I didn't want to take time off from work and have *that* disrupt my life."

Hospitalization rarely works when an anorexic is denying so much, because she honestly doesn't believe there's any sort of problem. In her mind, the whole world is just being a nag and a royal pain and that only angers and infuriates her. Being forced into the hospital is intensely threatening to the anorexic. It's a clear-cut battle: the anorexic against "Them." The hospital staff is trying to take away the only thing she's got. Consequently, an anorexic's main goal is to outsmart "Them," by "playing the game" and getting out.

"The first time I was hospitalized, I denied it completely," Chiara remarks. "*I* didn't have a problem — this guy was nuts!" So Chiara played along, gained weight, and got out.

"Every time I was hospitalized — and I was hospitalized a number of times — I would just eat and eat and eat, just to get out, and then I'd just lose the weight all over again," Chiara says. "I wasn't going to admit to having a problem—I couldn't. My mother always told me that anyone who saw a psychiatrist was nuts and no way was I going to fulfill my mother's prophecy. That's one thing that made it hard for me to ever get help.''

Alison's experiences were similar. She was forced into medical and psychiatric hospitals on numerous occasions and it was infuriating for her. "I remember being real angry at being force-fed and pulling out IVs and things like that," she says. "I was like, 'Don't *tell* me what to do, because it's the only thing I know *how* to do.'"

Alison sabotaged treatment a great deal in the hospital—pouring high-calorie liquid "sups" [liquid supplements] into potted plants and hiding food in drawers and shoes. But these ploys did not work in her favor. She quickly learned that she wouldn't be released from the hospital unless she was "a *good* patient" and gained weight. Hospitalization became a pointless recurring ritual for Alison. Whenever she'd go in for a "refeeding," that's all that would happen. "I'd go in, gain weight, and then I'd get back out and lose the weight," Alison says.

As Alison illustrates in this stage of acute denial when she's steadfastly determined to be anorexic, virtually nothing will change her mind. "In the hospital, I did things that were very counterproductive," admits Nancy. "I would get up very early in the morning during the time that the nurses were changing shifts and I would sneak outside and exercise. They were so busy hearing the morning report [an information update on the unit] that they didn't know what I was doing. So I would go outside the unit, out of the hospital, and go running around the parking lot."

Nancy loved getting away with it. "Part of the reason I did it was because it was beautiful, warm spring weather, and part of it was just plain old rebelliousness," she confesses with a laugh. "I was trapped inside and they wouldn't let me out. Also, part of it was to exercise and feel better about all that food I was eating. I got caught twice," Nancy adds with a grin, "but they figured I must be doing it other times. I was. I was also hiding food and putting food down my shirt front and in my pockets and then going in the room and throwing it out the window. Things like that.

"It was very strange," Nancy says reflectively. "Being in the hospital brought out every rebellious thing I'd ever felt. At home, I certainly don't act like that. I'm 42, and I was acting like I was about 12 when I was in the hospital. At home, I don't act that way, but in the hospital, having people giving me all this food and making me eat it, and sitting there watching me eat it, just brought out all of this resistance."

Not that Nancy is *totally* against hospital treatment programs. "If you are firmly committed to doing well, a good hospital program *can* work," she says. "But if you are at all ambivalent about it, there are a lot of loopholes. There are a lot of things you can do and get away with."

Learning the art of deception seems to be a major part of the initiation for first-timers in hospital eating disorder units. "You do, you learn a lot," says Nancy. "The first time I was hospitalized, I got a real education very quickly. Even though I didn't always *do* a lot there, I learned a lot about things and used them when the opportunities came."

Consequently, hospitalization is a very nebulous long-term solution, because it only works as well as the anorexic wants it to. Certainly, no one would advocate standing by and idly watching an anorexic starve herself to death. Yet the solution is definitely *not* to take away the one and only thing in her life she feels she has control over. It contradicts and defeats the entire purpose of what the anorexic needs to gain in recovery — positive coping skills to feel in charge of herself and her life.

"What the hospital does is make you feel very, very out-of-control and it's very demeaning," says Deborah. "You're treated almost as if you were a child. You go in there and the first thing they do is go through all of your clothes. So all of a sudden, you have this strange person going through your stuff and saying, 'We have to keep this in the nursing station and we have to keep that.' So right off the bat, that's there.

"Then they observe you going to the bathroom — every time you go to the bathroom — and *that* is very demeaning," Deborah says. "They monitor the meals — they monitor you pretty much the whole time you're on the unit. They monitor people because they feel like you *might* try to get away with something. Whether you do or don't, they *think* you're going to, which leads to a feeling of mistrust. It almost makes you *want* to try to get away with something.

And then at the same time, they're saying, 'Trust us, trust us, don't worry about how much food we're giving you.' It does make you *want* to do something. Just to get away with it.''

Deborah says she became bulimic after the first time she was hospitalized. "I was almost forced to be that way," she contends. "In the hospital, I was forced to eat a certain amount of calories — like 3,000 calories a day — which is a lot. I would just eat and eat and eat, just to get out, and then I couldn't do anything with it. So I'd go back in the hospital."

Eating disorder treatment programs that are grounded purely in changing an anorexic's behavior are ludicrous. Sure, they may "work" in the short-term (if "work" means injecting high-caloric liquids into her veins and forcing rapid weight gain). But if an anorexic is going to starve herself as soon as she leaves the hospital, what's the point? Long-term treatment programs, lasting a year or more in duration, seem to be the most positive and successful, as they provide intensive therapy and teach the anorexic new coping skills. However, these types of programs are more the exception than the rule.

Researcher Felicia Romeo (1986) criticizes many hospital treatment programs for being "too authoritarian" and behaviorally-oriented, focusing on the anorexic's weight gain, rather than her underlying psychological problems. Such reward-and-punishment programs miss the point entirely by emphasizing weight gain as the most important part of recovery.[1] They also lead the anorexic to conclude that the medical establishment doesn't really care about who she is as a person, only her poundage — as if she were nothing more than an object to be measured and weighed. The aim of such authoritarian programs — to harshly and rigidly control her, to "whip her into shape" and force her to obey (because "that's what she needs") — only lead her to rebel as soon as she gets the chance.

Heidi felt "pretty much obligated" to maintain her weight after she left the hospital. But she was counting the days until she'd leave home and could get back to losing weight. "I had to be weighed three times a week and if I went below my weight, things would be taken away from me," she remembers. "I would not be allowed to go bike riding or go for a walk. And then they kept pushing me up two pounds at a time. It was infuriating. Absolutely infuriating! I was just waiting until I graduated from high school to be free of all of that. Sure enough, the first semester in college, Heidi relapsed.

Hearing variations of this story over and over again pointed out the inadequacies of many hospital treatment programs. I'm sorry to report that few women I talked with said they were actually *helped* by a hospital treatment program. (Again, I must note that the programs that seemed to work best were long-term and focused first on underlying issues – an anorexic's emotional health and well-being – before tackling the issue of weight gain.)

Like several anorexic women, Jill had a real horror story to tell about the typical treatment program. "In the hospital," she says, "I had so many therapists that said, 'I don't want to deal with you because you're a chronic anorexic; you're going to go back in the hospital another time and another time. It's going to take you a hundred times before you're going to get better. I don't want to work with you. You don't *want* to get better.' How could you feel good about yourself when someone says *that* about you?"

Jill's treatment unit consisted of chemical abusers and other eating disordered patients. "Most of these other people that were in there were forced in there by the law or their parents. And there were some that were force-fed. There was one girl in there," Jill adds quietly, "and they finally said, 'Do you want to live or do you want to die? Do you want to be force-fed, or do you want to not be force-fed? It's up to you.' Because this girl – she just didn't want to do any of it. She wouldn't eat. They said, 'We don't want to deal with you anymore. You go to a halfway house. You go to a group home, because we can't do any more for you. If you don't want to live . . .'"

Jill says she didn't know where "that girl" was now, but they gave up on her.

The hospital had a "move 'em in, move 'em out" philosophy according to Jill. "Because of insurance, they wanted to get you out as quick as they could. So they'd get you up to your weight, and then you were out. They did a lot with the manic-depressive thing. They wanted to put you on drugs; they thought it was all keyed into drugs. 'Give her this drug and she'll be fine. She'll be all zombied out. She won't have any problems.' Well, take those drugs away and you're back to your old self. I didn't believe in that philosophy. I didn't want to spend the rest of my life on drugs."

Nancy, a three-time veteran of eating disorder treatment programs, questions the effectiveness of hospitalization. "I'm not sure that hospitalization is always effective because you can't really *deal* with your problems, if the problem is something at home," she says. "Or in my case, it had to do with my work. I couldn't do *that* in the hospital."

Nancy says she couldn't do much of *anything* in the hospital. "They don't allow you to move around very much," she says. "When I would walk around the hallway, they would nag me about it, or if I was swinging my feet, which I tend to do, they would clamp down on me. Then when we would go out on walks, I always walk very quickly—I'm a fast walker and they would get on me about that. When I was in there swinging my feet, someone was saying, 'Don't do that! You're burning calories!' Or if I was walking around, they said, 'Sit down! You're burning calories!'" Nancy felt like a prisoner. "Finally, I got out of the hospital, and the minute I stepped out the door," she grins, "I thought, 'Great! Now I don't have to eat anymore!'"

Hospital treatment programs haven't done a lot for Jessica either. "I've been hospitalized on and off—I'd hate to count how many times," Jessica says. "They've always tried to put weight on me, but it hasn't always been successful. They've always treated symptoms, but haven't gotten to the problem."

Jessica hated being locked up more than anything. "I *really* felt like a prisoner, especially on that 24-hour monitor," she says. "I'd get so jittery in there, because they confine you to a very small end of a hall, and you're not allowed to go to the other end. I just got too closed in. And then the nurse had to give me something. But it's just because you're restricted to this small area that contains a few sleeping rooms, a kitchen that's locked, and a small area with a TV. That's it. You've got no place to go and nothing to do. It's rough. They wouldn't even let us do situps. They caught one of the girls doing situps in the room one night and hollered at her. They wouldn't let us do anything like that. They checked on you during the night every 15 to 30 minutes. They opened your door and made sure that the bathroom was locked and they just had someone stationed there constantly. We had one phone between us twelve girls. It was *very* difficult.''

The last time she was hospitalized, Jessica believes she got everything out of it that she possibly could have, considering the frame of mind and denial she was in. ''It was just a routine,'' she says. ''Staying there wasn't going to change anything. Staying longer just made me more angry and I just would have refused to do more things.''

One of Jessica's pet peeves in the hospital was support group meetings. ''The girls were all struggling with the same thing, but once you've talked about it once, you don't need to talk about it a hundred million times,'' Jessica remarks. ''You just go to group after group after group 'til you're tired of talking about the same thing. In fact, we tell them that. You go to so many groups and you talk about the same things day in and day out. You have nutrition groups, community meetings, rap-up at night, your regular group during the day—you have family group and multi-family group—and they all talk about the same darn thing until you're tired of hearing about it.''

For many anorexics at this severe stage of addiction, group treatments can make the problem even worse. Competition is keen to be the thinnest in the room, which cancels any benefits of group interaction.

''Oh, the hospital was incredibly competitive,'' says Heidi. ''I was living on a ward with a bunch of other anorexics, and you just couldn't *eat* around them. Because they'd watch you, and you'd *know* they felt superior because you were eating and they weren't. If I was having something, they'd all want to come up and *smell* it,'' Heidi adds, ''and it just made me feel like, 'No, no, NO! If you're going to get anything out of this, you're going to have a *bite* of it! You're not going to get any enjoyment out of it and know that I'm eating it.' That made me angry. And they're just miserable people to live with. If you've ever been in the hospital, it gives you a whole new perspective. They'd congratulate you when they saw you'd put on a little weight. They'd say, 'Oh, you're really doing well; you're going forward,' and you'd be thinking inside, 'Oh, they're glad because I'm weighing more than they are now.'''

The intense competition among anorexic women isn't surprising. Competing against other women — particularly in regard to beauty ideals — is very much ingrained by our society. Close contact with other anorexics brings it all out.

"I never considered myself to be particularly competitive until I got into the hospital, and then I realized that yeah, I am," says Nancy. "After I had been in there a while, we got a new patient in who was, I thought, thinner than I was. And I just had a fit! She was about my same height and everything, and I was very surprised to find out that she actually weighed ten pounds more than I did."

Such intense competition prevents many acute anorexics from connecting with one another. "When I was very bad into anorexia, I heard about a support group, but I didn't want to go," Helena remembers. "I didn't want to meet other people with anorexia, because of the competition — 'That's *my* thing! I'm the *best* one; I need to be the thinnest!' In some stages, you can't take in other people," Helena concludes. "You're too obsessed with yourself, so you just feel they are all some kind of enemy."

Groups are not for the acute anorexic, nor do they appeal to them. Researchers Michele Siegel, Judith Brisman, and Margot Weinshel (1988) find that severely disturbed anorexics are so involved in their food and weight obsessions that they can't relate to other group members. It's extremely difficult for them to get outside of themselves and interact with others, since the primary focus of their attention is whether or not they are the thinnest person present. Consequently, they fail to benefit from mutual exchange in groups.[2]

In fact, severe anorexics often get sidetracked by other issues at support group meetings. "I attended a few meetings of the anorexic organization in Stockholm and I started to think it was almost okay to be anorexic after seeing the others in the group," Annett remarks. "I thought, 'You could probably be living like this, because others are doing it. It must not be so dangerous.' So I felt it was almost positive to have anorexia, to be like that. I felt like I didn't want to be well again."

Chronic anorexics who have no intention of recovering often

want to monopolize groups and discuss strategies and ideas for continuing their weight loss.

"Sometimes people want to get more attention from their husband, their family, from whoever, and sometimes they see the anorexia as a way of getting more attention," remarks Nancy. "Sometimes they feel like, 'Well, I have to get worse to get more attention. And I'm learning new tricks. This girl is talking about feeding her food to the dog; this girl's talking about putting the food in a napkin and throwing it out . . . maybe *I* can try that. Maybe I should do it more.' That kind of thinking — if you're already into it — can increase by participating in a group."

"If you're in a certain place and you see other women and you hear them, and this girl's real thin and she's talking about hitting the laxatives or hitting the diuretics, or 'All I eat for breakfast is one Cheerio' — if you're in a certain mood, sometimes that can influence you," Nancy adds. "You think, 'Well okay, that girl was thinner than I am and I want to be as thin as she is, so tomorrow, *I'll* only have one Cheerio or whatever.' Or, 'Well shoot, it wouldn't hurt to take a couple more laxatives — So-and-So takes ten at a time and she's alive to tell about it.' Sometimes I think people go in there and get worse because of hearing other people and thinking, 'Well I'm not as bad as she is.'"

The chronic anorexic *wants* to be "as bad as" the anorexic sitting next to her. *Worse* even. She *wants* to be "the best at being the thinnest." Maybe that's the most infuriating part of being hospitalized with other anorexics: reality hits. The one thing an anorexic thinks she has on everyone else — achieving thinness better than anyone — is gone because there's a whole ward of people doing the same thing she is.

"Everyone acts the same damn way you do," Chiara remarks. "When I'm anorexic, I have the same damn traits and behave the same damn way as any other anorexic. That's what starvation does to you. You act crazy and obsessed, just like all the other anorexics. So much for feeling unique and special."

Chapter 6

Choices

Sometimes, Chelsey feels anorexia nervosa is controlling *her.* "That's what's so scary about it," she says. "For a while there, I thought, 'This is great, I'm in so much control.' But then I thought, 'I'm not in control; it's controlling me. I'm really weak because I can't do anything about it.' But that's because I don't *want* to." That's why nothing changes — because deep down, the acute anorexic still wants to hang onto anorexia nervosa. She's caught up in denial and doesn't think she really has a problem — until finally, it starts to sink in. Like Chelsey, she realizes she's not in control after all. Anorexia nervosa is controlling *her.*

"I was sick from diuretics," Nancy recalls. "I was taking laxatives heavily, and I had to stay home from work a couple of times because I was sick and I couldn't get out of bed. Then I started to realize, 'Maybe I *have* lost control and the disease is really controlling me.'"

The obsessive thinking was a signal. "The more you do it, the more you become obsessed," Nancy says. "*That* was something I *knew* wasn't normal and I felt it was something I couldn't control. It just came whether I wanted it to or not, so I felt that was very much controlling me, too."

Anorexics start to realize that the control they think they have is only an illusion. "I think [the illusion] is sure, you seem to be in control on the outside," says Jill, "but subconsciously, there are a lot of things you've put in little boxes inside your head and said, 'They're okay for now.' Or, 'They're not as important as the other things right now.' Or, 'I don't really know the answer; I'm going to give it some more time.' Then all of a sudden," Jill says, "you realize that somebody's knocking on your door inside of you, saying, 'Hey, hey — you really aren't paying attention to me. I've got a problem in here! Listen to me! *LISTEN TO ME!*' And it starts tearing everything else apart and those things that you had under control are no longer in control.

"Your mind starts playing games," says Jill. "Being at a low weight compounds it. It adds to your inability to focus the stress. And then it snowballs. When you get down to my weight, it's really serious. My mind is not functioning the way it should. I know that. It's a feeling that you're impatient. You're fed up with waiting. You're tired of things the way they are, but you don't know what the answer is. You want something to change, but you don't know how to change it. Mine's not so much the eating as it is the exercising. After the exercising kicks in . . . it's like tightening a rubber band to the point where it will break."

When Jill was released from the hospital, she was thirty pounds heavier than she was going in. But weight was all she gained. She had no resources with which to cope. "Everything was just swimming around," Jill says. "It was like I didn't feel anything. I was at the right weight of what I should be. I had all the physical capabilities. But I had no idea of what to do next."

Jill says she knew before she went in the hospital that the solution wasn't simply a matter of gaining weight. "I could do that any day — gain weight," she says. "It's how do I feel about myself? Who am I as a person? [The hospital staff could make me] say affirmations every day up the wazoo, but it was not going to work because I was not going to believe it.

"Then there was my father," Jill recalls. "'Jill, you look *great*. You've got it all together; let's go out and conquer the world!' And I thought, 'You don't know what it's like, Daddy. I hate myself! I hate myself right now more than anything. I don't know anything about myself. I am so depressed!' I wasn't happy, and yet everyone thought I *should* be happy. No one knew I hadn't even begun to tackle the problems. The only thing I knew how to do was exercise and restrict food. And I got depressed. I didn't have a sense of worthiness. Or an inner voice. Or a sense that there was really anything to me. I felt empty. And I wanted to die."

Like many women, Alison had to hit bottom before she was able to recognize and admit she had a problem. "Some of my friends said they were afraid that I was going to die. This one friend kept saying she'd never seen anyone *that* thin, and she was just scared to death to be around me," Alison says. "That's the only real reaction I got."

But *Alison* still didn't think she had a problem. "It came to the point where the group of friends that I'd been hanging out with just couldn't deal with me anymore," she remembers. "I only had one person I could talk to. I was so depressed and she started telling me, 'You're anorexic. You're anorexic, and that could be a lot of why you're not having friends and you're finding things very difficult.' She called an eating disorder unit, or a hotline or something, and got some information for me. About the same time, I got really dehydrated and I was in the hospital at school—it was a little infirmary-type thing. I remember her bringing the information she'd gotten down to me, and at the same time, the nurses were telling me, 'You're so dehydrated you're not going to be able to go back to class.' And I felt like everything in the world was falling apart. I *had* to do something."

Finally, it gets to the point where there's no other choice left. "I got so obsessed with losing weight that I wasn't interested in anything else," says Monica. "I was very unhappy. I realized that this was sick—my thoughts were sick. You can't live for losing weight. It's not normal. I realized that and I was so depressed. Then I realized, 'I hate myself! I need help.'"

Brenda says she finally hit the point when she was tired of being in so much pain. "My whole life revolved around food," she says. "When I got up in the morning, I would eat, and then the only thing I could think about for the whole morning was lunch. Then after lunch, the only thing I could think about was dinner. My evenings were spent chasing food, and that's how I felt—like I was chasing it. I just started to feel crazy. I didn't feel it then, but now I know— it's like trying to fill a hole in yourself."

The anorexic's mission of starvation—to reach the ultimate state of thinness—can never fill the emptiness. When everything else is stripped away, the anorexic must finally make a choice of whether to live or die.

Jessica is still trying to make that choice. "When they told me in the hospital that I was going to die, I was kind of happy," she says, "because I knew I was going to be with my children. And that's what I wanted most of all." Yet the balance tips toward life on other days. "I *think* I want to [live]," Jessica says, "but I'm not positive. Those down days are really bad. They're really down. As low as I can go. And I don't sometimes know how to get me out of them. Sometimes I don't *want* to come out of them and it worries me because there *is* a lot I still want to do in life. But there's a lot I want to do that I'll never be able to, too. And I have to divide those and get in my mind what's real and what isn't. And I haven't done that yet."

Jessica sometimes scares herself. "I find myself sleeping more now and napping, which I never used to do, and that worries me," she says, "because I have a feeling like I'm getting more and more depressed. But I don't like being on medication. So I don't know how to fight the difference. I don't know what the happy medium is on that." It's frustrating because Jessica has seen every therapist in her area over the past five years. "I couldn't get along with any of them," she says. "I don't know what's going to make a definite change. I don't know what's going to change my mind around."

Monica is convinced that breaking through the denial is the only way to make that change, to take the first step toward recovery. "You have to *want* to get well, to *really* want it," Monica says. "And it takes a lot of time sometimes. It's only been in the last year that I've stopped lying to myself. Even though I admitted six-and-a-half years ago that I was ill, it's taken time not to lie to myself. Because you can lie, even though you *know* the truth. You can deny it; you can tell yourself, 'Today—I'm not ill today. No, no, no, no, I have no problems. Okay, okay, I didn't eat last night. But it's okay. I'm just like anybody else.' You think *someone else* is anorexic, but not you. It's hard to recognize it in yourself."

Recognizing and admitting anorexia nervosa is the first step to recovery. An anorexic must also *choose* to get better and want it more than anything, because if she's lying to herself, nothing will change. She could spend the rest of her life just going through the motions—spinning through the revolving door of hospitals, therapists, nutritionists, and on and on—all meaningless exercises in futility.

Annett is struggling through the process of admitting she needs help to recover from anorexia. "I'm *starting* to admit I have a problem and know I need to get help, but I have a great deal of anxiety every time I eat," she says. "They want to keep me here in the hospital until they see I can manage myself, until they see I can stay home and manage the food. But it's not possible for me to go home and be alone right now. I would never be able to manage that. Because if I were to go home right now, I wouldn't be eating."

Recognizing that anorexia *is* a problem is the most difficult part. "Sometimes I feel it's pretty hopeless," says Annett. "Sometimes I'm ready to give up. As soon as I start to feel a little better, I think, 'Oh, this will be okay. I think I can fix it myself.' Then I want to get out of here. But I know I can't. It takes a long time to get to the point where you ask for help—to admit you have it."

It's not easy for an anorexic to see what she's doing: desperately trying to fill the emptiness in her life. It's hard to see anorexia nervosa objectively when stuck in it and it's difficult to realize the other options. It's hard to see that you *can* be happy, that you don't have to live a life ruled by obsessions, hating yourself with a vengeance.

Sometimes it takes another person who truly cares to jolt an anorexic out of her tunnel vision. In Heidi's case, it was an unconditionally accepting friend. "I met Katie my freshman year of college, and she just took an active interest in me," Heidi remembers with a smile. "It was the first time in a long time that I'd gotten into a sincere and mutual friendship, and that just took my attention away from myself. I think that helps a lot, because as an anorexic, you're so self-centered and self-scrutinizing."

At the time, Heidi says she was desperate to have a friend like Katie. "I remember wishing I just had one friend I could go to at any time and say anything. And Katie was very unconditional and very accepting, right from the start. I remember one day, we went to a restaurant together, and I said, 'Oh, I'm not going to have anything,' and Katie said, 'Well, I am.' To me, it was just unthinkable that someone could be comfortable eating while the other one wasn't—to be watched while you were eating—but it didn't bother

her in the least. Katie just wanted to hear my story—what anorexia was and how it was affecting me. She wanted to hear it all—and she was eating and it wasn't bothering her at all. I just thought that was great."

Katie *inspired* Heidi to recover. "Katie, I think, has had every drop of self-respect and self-esteem that she's needed since she was about 12," laughs Heidi. "And she's very open, talking about anything about herself—what she's afraid of, what she likes, what she has a right to in any situation. I've learned a lot from her."

A supportive person who accepts an anorexic just the way she is, has been a pivotal element in recovery for many women. Chiara credits her therapist for helping her to see beyond anorexia. "Sticking it out with one therapist and building a relationship and bonding and trusting him has been so important in my recovery," remarks Chiara. "The first time I met him, I didn't like him because he seemed so intimidating. But something in me knew that it was all right. Things started to click and happen."

Chiara admits it took nearly a year and a half to trust her therapist. "I was in the hospital twice and he was the director there, so that helped even more to build trust, and for him to know me even more," Chiara says. "But that's scary, too, because I sit back and think, 'My God, this guy *really* knows me, like no one else knows me.' He knows what I'm thinking sometimes. But he knows me enough to be able to counteract my unhealthy self."

Helena's psychiatrist has been a crucial support in her recovery as well. "I had been seeing my psychiatrist for ten years, and this past Tuesday was our last meeting," she says. "Over the years, I sometimes went once, sometimes five days a week, depending on how I felt. Sometimes, I just talked about how fat I was, even though I wasn't. But he was someone I could count on. It was a place that I could be safe, without any demands. I could be myself. It was the only place I felt accepted. No matter what, he would still be there for me. It *has* taken a lot of time," Helena says. "Perhaps if I had done other things, it would have gone faster. But I'm not sure. Because first, I had to accept that I *needed* help."

Seeking professional help is a monumental risk for many. But with the right therapist—one with a feminist perspective, who understands the complex pressures and demands for a woman in our society — the payoffs can be tremendous.

"My therapist has been the most important part of my recovery," says Monica. "Before, I didn't feel I had any contact with people. I had friends, but I didn't feel I could reach them. I was isolated, and felt that nobody cared for me. They *did*, but I didn't feel it. So I started isolating myself. But when I met my therapist, I felt that she *saw* me, she was interested in me, and she cared. I found this one person who could be a bit of a mother maybe — a stable person, who I could say anything to, and rely on.

"I think I was *ready* to recover," Monica adds. "It's been awful, because I've been very sick. I've been in therapy for six-and-a-half years. I was really bad. I couldn't work. I was totally depressed and food-obsessed. But I'm really impressed that she held onto me, because even my mother said to me, 'You're a hopeless case. You'll *never* recover.' Even though I was so obsessed with food, I still could work with my therapist. She's not interested in weight or anything. When I go down too much, she tells me, 'Well if you don't stop, you'll end up in the hospital.' But she gives me so much love that I don't go down. Because I know somebody cares.

"She [therapist] doesn't tell me what I feel," Monica adds. "If I tell her something I have felt, not here and now, but something that happened yesterday, she doesn't go on and talk a lot about it. She just says, 'Yes, it's okay.' She's very accepting of *my* feelings, *my* thoughts. She thinks that *my* feelings are the important ones, my thoughts about my feelings. She doesn't think she knows better, *I* know better. I am the expert of *me* and my feelings. I have to have someone like that, and this therapist is like that. She's accepting me, so I can accept myself because I see that someone else does."

Monica believes you need love and acceptance more than anything in recovery. "Sometimes it can be a friend or a therapist," she says, "but just knowing they're there, no matter what, and they love you anyway. You need to know you're good as you are. You're not good because you have high marks and things like that. You're good, even if you just sit for a whole day on the sofa, you are still a fabulous person because everybody deserves to be loved. That's what you have to realize."

In addition to her therapist's unconditional encouragement and support, Robin feels her therapist has been a role model for her. "I've gained a sense of trust in myself by learning from my therapist's example in a lot of ways—from the way that she has handled certain situations, because I saw her in the hospital, standing up for her beliefs."

Robin's therapist has taught her a powerful lesson: that women can be powerful and can assert strong convictions and beliefs. "I view her [my therapist] as an individual, as a person having opinions and standing behind those opinions, and it's just had a big impact on me," Robin says. "And I've often felt she's the one person who really understands me."

Of course, letting another person in is very scary. "The thing is, I just can't trust anybody else," says Annett. "I don't dare make any contacts because I don't dare show who I really am. I'm ashamed of myself and afraid of making a fool of myself. I want to be perfect all the time. I'm afraid of being disappointed, that other people will let me down and because of that, I don't dare give of myself."

Annett is afraid to get close to anyone, because she fears that once they see "the *real* Annett," they'll abandon her. Like many women recovering from anorexia, Annett views the world through a conditional lens, as in, "If they see who I really am—a flawed person—they won't want anything to do with me." (Once anorexic women recover, however, they realize that *that's* what makes them lovable: they're human; they slip up at times; they're not perfect, and they make mistakes just like everyone else.)

It *is* difficult to risk letting another see your vulnerabilities. Annett's fear is her greatest obstacle; still, she craves unconditional acceptance from another human being more than anything. "If I should get anyone to like me, either a very good friend that I could talk to about anything, or if I could find a boy that would really love me . . . if I would have that, then I wouldn't think so much about anorexia," she says. "That is what I really want. I want to be loved and feel that I'm accepted as I am. But I don't dare because I'm afraid that they will react negatively or say no, and that they wouldn't want me at all. That's what I really want inside. That's what my whole soul is craving for, but at the same time, I'm afraid." Annett must realize she's not alone. There are others on the same path who care and want to help. She doesn't have to suffer in silence and isolation.

Helena strongly believes in support groups, but only if an anorexic truly wants to be well. "If you don't want to be well, if you want to keep where you are, then it's not the right time to go to a group," Helena says. "Because then you will be afraid of other people who *are* getting better. You have to come to a point where you *want* to be well. You can't lie to yourself."

It took years of therapy before Monica felt ready to attend a support group. "Therapy was very important for me first because it's easier — it was for me — to open myself to one person, one who listens and sits there, than to be in a group where you have to take responsibility and all that. It's only been in the last year that I've been able to go to the group. I went two years ago, but I was so ill that I couldn't . . . I wasn't paranoid, but I felt that nobody liked me, and I felt lonely. It was scary. It takes several [meetings] to feel comfortable and feel yourself. But now, I hear other people's stories and I see that I have the same problems and very much the same feelings, too. And so I realized, yes, I have this problem and there are lots of others who have it, and I'm not alone."

Even if it's scary in the beginning — even if the anorexic is too afraid to say anything at all — support groups can be very comforting (*if*, of course, she's ready to be receptive to others). At least she knows she's not alone.

"I like to listen," says Chelsey. "It's real interesting to hear other people. I've felt, 'Wow, that person thought the same thing *I* did and I thought I was crazy!' That's what I like about it, just listening to other people."

Jessica has met friends in her weekly group that have been a tremendous support in her recovery. Since the group members are all waging the same battle, she feels comfort in knowing they understand the ups and downs. "I think right now, for the first time in my life, having friends to talk to has really helped," says Jessica. "They understand. It's just a long recovery and knowing I'm not alone has helped."

For Nancy as well, meeting with others who understand anorexia continues to be an important part of her recovery. In fact, her support group helped her break through her denial, to realize what she was doing to herself and to finally seek treatment.

"Finally, when I was in the support group, I heard other women talk about weighing themselves all the time," says Nancy, "and not eating; or eating very little, or obsessing about what they *did* eat, or obsessing about the number of calories. And I thought, 'Well I don't worry too much about the calories. I *know* what I'm eating, so I don't obsess or worry about it. I *know* how many calories it has.' That's because I had restricted my diet to so few things."

"I kept going to the support group, and then one day, the group leader took me aside," Nancy recalls. "I finally talked about myself a little bit, and at that point, I had gotten down to about 78 or 76, so she took me aside and suggested I talk to a doctor in charge of admissions at a local hospital. I had been in psychiatric therapy — I was going once a week to another doctor who didn't deal with eating disorders, and he and I had talked about anorexia a couple of times, but he didn't put too much emphasis on it. So I told the group leader, 'I'm *in* therapy now. I don't really need to go see someone else.' But she kind of twisted my arm a bit. So finally I went to see this doctor, and he took one look at me, and said, 'You need to be hospitalized.' And I said, 'No, no, I don't have time!' We were in the middle of refinancing our house and we were trying to do all that, and I said, 'I don't have time. I work! When would I have time to go into the hospital? I have some sick leave, but I don't want to be using it all up for this!'"

Nancy finally broke down and told her husband after her talk with the group leader. "I mentioned to my husband, 'Well, you know I may have anorexia, but I'm not sure, that's why I've got to go see this doctor," she remembers. "The woman who runs the support groups seems to think I should.' And he said, 'Well, you look all right to me.' And I said, 'Well, I have kind of lost a lot of weight.' So then I took off my clothes and all that, and he could see."

Gradually, the support group helped Nancy admit she had a problem and not to be ashamed of it. "Through the support group, I learned that maybe it was okay, that I was not as abnormal as I thought I was if I had certain thoughts or did certain things," she says. "I began to realize that I didn't have to beat myself up about it — that other people do the same thing."

Nancy says she's learned many other coping skills through the group as well. "I think I've learned a lot about how to handle myself and how to handle other people more, too — to be more diplomatic, more tactful, and also more open," Nancy remarks. "I was never very open before. I've learned an *awful* lot about other people, and myself, too. I always used to keep pretty much to myself, so I didn't know a lot about others because I didn't have much contact with them in an intimate way. I was always very distanced. But it's been a real revelation to see and hear other people going through a lot of the same things and realize I'm not alone. I listen to people and think, 'Yeah, yeah, what she's saying, I have felt that, I have done that, and felt real stupid about it.' Well she's saying the same thing and she looks all right. She's a nice girl. So I must not be crazy after all."

For several women I talked with, support groups grounded in spirituality have been an important strength throughout their recoveries. One such program is Overeaters Anonymous (OA), a 12-step program that offers group meetings in larger metropolitan areas for recovering anorexics.

"OA has given me hope," says Linda. "My sponsor has been so wonderful and supportive, and I've thought, 'If she can do it, so can I.' And it's so nice to be able to call her when I feel I need to talk to someone. My faith in a Higher Power gives me strength and perspective," Linda adds, "especially when I find myself in a lonely or self-pitying mood. When I'm able to see that what I'm experiencing is part of the grand scheme of life — that there's always a lesson for me to learn — I'm able to see things more objectively, and at my best moments, to not be quite so hard on myself."

Other women, however, mentioned that they were uncomfortable with such 12-step programs because of the idea of "giving away their power, their control to a God." "Twelve-step programs make me feel I'm not in control anymore," says Alison. "They don't work for me."

While 12-step programs such as OA play a key role for certain women, I must point out that the program treats food in much the same way as Alcoholics Anonymous (AA) — on which its tenets are based — treats alcohol. Granted, you can live without alcohol. But not food. That's where the ideology gets a little twisted. OA stresses "abstaining" from certain foods, such as those with sugar and flour. "Abstaining" seems to be a different word for the same concept: "restricting," or more simply, "dieting." To many, it seems that a program which promotes dieting simply carries on the issues and obsessions a woman recovering from anorexia nervosa is trying to steer away from.

Still, Brenda finds the program works for her. "In OA, they call it your Higher Power and some people call it God or whatever, but I think it's that part of you that knows what is best for you and cares about you," she says. "And that part of me does not want me to starve myself because that's not good for *me* — it's self-destructive. It's that part somewhere inside that wants what's best for *me*.

"When I was into my food and everything, I just remember feeling so alone," Brenda remarks. "And now, I know I'm not alone anymore. By connecting with other people who cared, I found the strength to do what's best for me. I let go of my eating disorder because I realized it was only destroying me, hurting me. I chose life instead."

Chapter 7

Changes

Helena woke up in a hospital bed at ground zero. "I was in intensive care, almost dying, because I had lost so much weight. It was very close," she says. After intravenous tube feedings, Helena began to regain her senses. "I remember when I got nutrition, my first thought was, 'I'm thinking again! I have thoughts!'" she remembers. "Then it was, 'I can stand on my legs!' Then I felt like a pioneer, going into the mountains and thinking. Lying there in the hospital room, I was by myself and did a lot of thinking."

That was the first step for Helena in exploring the issues underlying her struggle with anorexia nervosa. She needed to return to a safer, more stable weight before she regained the physical, mental, and emotional faculties to delve beneath the symptom. But even then, it wasn't so easy. First, Helena had to let go of some of the control. "I wasn't really prepared to gain the weight," she admits. "Because when you eat a little bit, suddenly you feel the hunger. And then I was afraid. So I said, 'Now I must get out of the hospital! I must get out and start controlling again!' I thought I had lost the control because I felt the hunger. So I left the hospital and then it was another phase. Then you are having nutrition—you can think—but that's even worse, because then all the feelings and anxiousness come back, and you have to deal with all of that."

Gaining weight is *not* the difficult part. Dealing with the thoughts and feelings that come racing to the surface is. Because that's when the recovering anorexic starts feeling out of control. "I've *tried* to gain before and I'd go up a couple of pounds and then I'd freak out and go back down," Chelsey remarks. "It's just knowing that I was gaining and feeling out of control. I guess maybe that's a signal that I'm just not ready to gain yet."

Getting over the resistance to weight gain *is* a tough proposition. But the recovering woman must begin to trust . . . and let go of the control, even if it's just a little bit at first. Chiara remembers how difficult it was. "Even when I recognized that I *did* have a problem, it was still hard, because I didn't realize how much I would have to give up," she says. "In the hospital, I hated being incarcerated, being threatened with IVs, and having no freedom, because I felt like I was being abused again. But when I started trying to let go of some of my control and trying to trust the dietician and the doctor and what they were saying, I was able to reach out for their help. Once I was a little bit nourished and could think and concentrate, it was easier because I was ready to deal with the issues."

As with many anorexic women, exploring the causes underlying anorexia was a very painful process for Chiara. "During the six months I was in the hospital, I had to constantly separate issues of abuse and issues of food," Chiara explains. "I was always project-ing on the staff at the hospital. I'd see a quality of my mother in the nurse, so therefore, I would react to the nurse like I would react to my mother. I wouldn't trust her. So I had to learn to separate those two things. Being in the hospital made it harder, because I didn't *have* any control and I felt really trapped. I was *forced* to deal with the issues."

That's the scariest part. So many feelings and thoughts that the anorexic has tried so hard to deny and numb are suddenly exposed. It's as if a vein has opened and the feelings come surging out. Sud-denly, these women don't know what to do with it all.

For Annett, being in the hospital is terrifying because there's nowhere to run. "At home, I can hide away—escape," she says. "Here I have to eat and face my problems. When I eat, I feel dis-gusted, and here, I have to face my emotions. When I stop eating, my anxiety disappears. But here in the hospital, I don't have that choice. I have to sit down and really question myself." That takes a lot of courage. Facing the pain is never easy. "When I start to examine myself and ask myself what I'm doing, I get very de-pressed," admits Annett. "But that is what I really need to bring up. I have to face those issues. And I'm trying to understand why I'm doing this. I want to find a reason, so I can do something about it and change. But although that's what I want to do, it's very difficult, because I have discovered a lot of things about myself—many things that I had never thought about before. Because whenever I have had to face something that was difficult, I've denied it completely, as if it didn't exist.''

One of the major changes anorexics must make in recovery is breaking through the denial and uncovering the causes of the problem. They must explore their thoughts and feelings to understand why they have been starving themselves. Slowly, they will start to gain insight into why they turned away from food when anxious, confused, and angry—and what they were trying to say through anorexia nervosa.

Nancy experienced two hospital stays before she was ready to explore the underlying issues. "The first time I went into the hospital, all these people were sitting around talking about their feelings," Nancy remembers. "And talk, talk, talk, talk all day long. Somebody would ask me things, and I'd say, 'I'm fine, I'm fine. Well, I have this thing about not eating, but otherwise, I'm fine.' It took them a long time to break through the barriers with me."

Nancy says she fought gaining weight "tooth and nail," every step of the way. "I gave them a harder time in the beginning," she says. "I had a few problems with eating meals, and when the first few pounds went on, I exploded around that. To me, that was the worst thing in the world. My weight was just going to fly up from there. I absolutely disagreed with their range. Who were *they* to tell me that I should weigh 130 pounds?! I did not need to weigh that much, and I would argue it—usually every ten pounds. When I would get over the 100 mark or the 110 mark, it would be a major issue all over again."

Trusting the hospital staff was difficult for Leslie as well. "I was forced to eat in the hospital," she says, "and I was totally anxious. There was just no way out of it. I *had* to eat. But for me, the hospital was a very supportive environment. Still, I was just really anxious. And it was scary, too. I would think, 'Oh, you're going to make me fat. Oh no!' And they would say, 'You have to trust us. We're not going to make you fat.' They did a lot of reality testing like, 'If you were walking down the street, do you think people would stop and say, 'Boy, is that woman overweight?' And I'd say, 'Well, your sample on the street—that's a biased sample.' So they had to work with me a lot before I was willing to trust and realize that I wasn't fat and they weren't going to make me fat."

Reality testing helped Alison as well, in seeing herself more accurately and recognizing the need to gain weight. "In one hospital I was in, they did a lot of testing of perceptions and things," she says. "There were all sorts of things they did, instead of just standing us in front of the mirror and saying, 'Look at you! Look at you!' Like body tracing — we'd lie down on paper and they would measure our arms and make a circle just to show us. They also took Polaroids, so we'd be seeing ourselves not from a mirror, but actual pictures. That was one thing that made me start realizing what I looked like."

When Alison began to realize she was extremely thin — *too* thin — and needed to gain weight, she was ready to move on. She began to explore the deeper underlying issues: what was *really* going on and why she had turned to anorexia nervosa in order to cope.

Helena believes anger and self-hatred lie at the core of her struggle with anorexia. "All of the anger, I put on myself," she says. "I *hated* myself. I had a period — oh, it wasn't good — when I was so angry with myself that in the evening, when I was going to bed, I felt so many anxieties inside of me that I would hit my head on the wall. So I had bumps everywhere on my head. The wall was in my parents' home, and I had a piece of cloth on the wall because it was a little bit cold. When I was moving from my parents' house and we took it down, there was a big hole. That was from my head. So all of the anger was there."

The underlying issue for Chiara was buried pain from enduring years of physical and sexual abuse. Anorexia nervosa was a way for her to escape, to numb the feelings, to block out the pain, to try to forget. "To be vulnerable in my house was to be exposed," says Chiara. "To be weak around my family meant that you would be hurt even more, so I had to squash my feelings. I couldn't acknowledge that feelings were there. As I grew up, I didn't know what I was feeling, so I put in its place, 'fat' — 'I'm fat, I'm fat, I'm fat.' I never felt anything. As soon as an emotion would spring forth, I'd hop on the scale."

Obsessions with food, weight, and thinness also served as an escape for Alison — to numb her feelings. "When I was in the hospital, I had a tendency—like when doctors would ask me how I felt—I would always tell them that I didn't *know*," she says. "I had no idea what I was feeling. I *wasn't* hungry; I *wasn't* depressed or anything like that. I just had a problem with food. I felt I needed to control everything, to make things just right. I thought, 'The only way I can control everything in my life is to control my eating.' So I've had to learn to separate food and weight from what I'm thinking and feeling. That's probably been one of the hardest things, because for me, it *is* a big control."

One of the most helpful strategies Alison found in working through the control issue, is exploring her deepest thoughts and feelings by keeping a journal. "I have a new obsession—keeping a journal," she says with a laugh. "And that has helped me a lot, because I think one of my major problems was communication. I seem to be able to write down a lot of the feelings I couldn't say. I try to write as often as I can, just whatever my feelings are, and that really helps," Alison says. "When you put it down on paper, it's not so overwhelming. Trying to connect my feelings and food has probably been *the* most important thing in my recovery, and writing has really helped me with that."

Writing is a key strategy that many anorexic women have used to gain awareness and insight into the underlying issues. Some write out the thoughts and feelings that surface in therapy, the hospital, and through discussions with other recovering anorexics. Others write whatever comes to mind through self-exploration, introspection, and self-study.

The important point is to be uncensored—to write whatever springs to mind, whatever needs to get out. It's not supposed to be a perfect, eloquent essay. It's just for the writer and that's all it needs to be. Recovering women must be able to write whatever pops into their minds, whatever issues they're grappling with, whatever they want to vent. As the anorexic begins to get in touch with these thoughts and feelings, her personal struggle will begin to make sense . . . in time.

Another strategy women have used in exploring the meaning of their struggle with anorexia is simply sharing their thoughts and feelings with others. "It's been through my therapist, through therapy," says Monica. "And also by thinking, writing, and very much, by communicating with others. Socializing—just *daring* to-socialize—has been very important for me. Then I see myself in other people and I realize I'm not as bad as I thought. Because others tell me they like me, when before, I thought I was some kind of—not a monster, really—but awful and boring and everything. When you dare to socialize with people, they teach you lots more than you can ever get to yourself."

Monica believes that getting outside of herself and making contact with others has been crucial in her recovery. "You can't sit alone on the sofa and just think, 'Who am I?'" she says with a laugh, "because I tried that and it didn't work out. Instead of just sitting and thinking too much, it's very good to write or paint or get outside of yourself in some way. If something bothers you, just write or draw and express what you're feeling. Don't worry about whether it's perfect; just write or draw or paint whatever's in your head."

Connecting with others through groups helped Leslie break through her wall of feelings. "In the hospital, I learned a lot of different ways to get in touch with the feelings I had and to express my feelings," Leslie says. "Through art and writing and movement therapy, I began to understand my pain. The hospital was a very supportive environment and very intensive with the different groups on feelings, assertive communication, group therapy, occupational therapy, dance therapy, art therapy. My day was very structured—and I needed that. But I think the most helpful thing was the support."

Leslie's hospital treatment program was exemplary in helping her to gain new coping skills. Since she left the hospital (it had been nearly two years when I spoke with her), her progress has been steady. "I've had some dips," Leslie says, "but for the most part, I've been moving along. I kept the therapist that I had in the hospital, which really helped, because he's an excellent therapist. I've been with him almost three years and we've been working on a lot of the issues. It's been problematic at times, but not to the point that it was when I went into the hospital."

The reality for many women is that progress is *not* always steady, however. Recovering from anorexia nervosa—particularly for women with a chronic pattern of anorexic behaviors—is a long and arduous process, with triumphs and sometimes, setbacks.

Even though Robin "graduated" from a long-term treatment program for anorexia, she hadn't broken through her denial when she was released. In the hospital, she'd concentrated her energies on being "a good patient" to please the hospital staff. Robin did everything she was supposed to, to earn more privileges and get out sooner.

"As far as the eating was concerned, I was pretty cooperative," Robin remembers. "I would go ahead and eat the meals, whereas a lot of people didn't. And I would go to the groups and things like that. I just tried to do whatever they wanted me to do in order to gain more and more privileges, because that's the kind of program it was. And so by being 'good,' I continued advancing up and getting more and more freedom. But at the same time, I was not revealing a lot of my obsessions," she admits, "so they were not able to help me with certain things. I was afraid that the doctors and the other patients would judge me. I was so much into denial with myself—that would cause me to hold back a lot of the time."

Consequently, when Robin was released from the hospital, she relapsed into anorexia, which is completely understandable. In the hospital, she had only gained weight, not the coping skills needed to handle real life.

Robin had played the game. She had to be at her goal weight— 130 pounds—to be released from the hospital. "Then I quickly went down to 105 pounds," she says. "It was because of the stress. When I came out, I was suddenly out of the security of the hospital and I thought that being released from the hospital meant that I could handle the world again. But inside, I *wasn't* ready to handle the world. And after being in the hospital for so long, I came out and discovered that the same issues were still out there—the relationships with people, my career, family problems—it was all still there. It was just a lot of pressure and I crumbled under it. My way of asking for help from others and saying to people, 'Hey, all of you—this is going on and I don't know what to do about it,' was to restrict."

Robin says it was a paradox. She was trying to communicate how much pain she was in through anorexia nervosa. "I would nonverbally say things," she says, "but people don't always know what you're trying to say to them unless you verbally say it."

Consequently, therapy has been crucial in helping Robin to delve into these issues, and also, to learn to trust others. "It's been a difficult experience for me to get close to someone," she says. "I have always had a problem with trust, so it was scary at first. But by opening up to my therapist, I've been able to see that people are not always out to hurt me in some way."

Through the recovery process, Robin has learned to get in touch with who she is. "I've learned that I am an individual, that I have feelings and opinions and I'm entitled to have my own feelings and opinions — *and* to express them," she says. "And if somebody else does not agree, that does *not* make me wrong. I will not disintegrate if somebody disagrees with what I say."

Robin has learned to stand up for her convictions in this stage of self-exploration. "I've learned to express my feelings to another person, and that has really made a difference," she says. "If I disagree with the way something is done or somebody else's opinion, I've learned to go ahead and stand up for what *I* think is right, to just express that. Afterward, I feel so much better. Even if it goes their way, no matter what the results are, just the fact that I said how I feel — it's been really important for me."

Yet perhaps the most difficult part of finding out "who you are" is that it's an entirely new way-of-being. Instead of simply doing, saying and being whatever "they" want, a recovering anorexic must begin to rely on herself and her own inner guidance. No one can discern what feels right, what she believes in, and what she wants out of life, but the recovering individual.

Alison remembers how difficult it was in the beginning. "I used to *always* do whatever anyone told me to do. I always tried to please everybody. I tried to do whatever they wanted me to do just to make them like me," Alison says. "But as I began recovering, I had to learn to recognize what *I* want and need. I think that's been the first step toward being assertive and getting what I want. Because I don't think before, I even knew. I just did whatever anyone told me to do."

Helena had to learn to let go of being the "Superwoman" — perfect in every way and always "on," all the time. "Before, I didn't know who I was," Helena says. "I just wanted to be . . . so that other people would be satisfied. I had to learn to let go of all the demands from everywhere, and also my demands from myself to be so perfect and be the best."

In her book, *Addiction to Perfection*, Jungian analyst Marion Woodman (1982) observes that the anorexic woman is so busy doing and achieving, that she loses touch with the other side of herself—her deepest self, her "inner life . . . which gives meaning to symbols and conversely the symbols which give meaning to life."[1]

The anorexic woman has alienated and blocked off her inner self. She doesn't know what it's like to laugh and play, to be spontaneous, creative, and carefree. She doesn't know what it means to goof off, to be free from all worries, to take a "wait-and-see" attitude toward life. "Going with the flow" is an alien concept to her, because she's made a habit of being serious, controlled and driven. She doesn't know what it means to simply be herself. Because she can't let go. The control she thinks she has over herself and her life is only an illusion. The paradox is, to truly *gain* control—personal power—in her life, she must first let go and let her heart—her inner self—be the guide.

Jill is trying, really trying. "One of the biggest issues for me right now is feeling like I'm doing something that's unique in my life," Jill says, "that nobody else can do, that nobody else *will* do, that nobody else *wants* to do—because it's not them. It's what *I'm* here to do. And I'm trying to find out what that is."

When a recovering anorexic finds out who she is, the rest follows. She begins to realize her likes and dislikes, her preferences and opinions, and then she begins to define her boundaries. "When I was anorexic, I felt all these demands from other people, but I never knew what *I* wanted," says Kelly. "So the first step was learning to ask, 'What do *you* want, Kelly?'—before I did anything."

Kelly had to learn to acknowledge her feelings and her opinions—her inner guidance. She's learned to listen, and act accordingly. She needed to learn to stand up for herself and her beliefs, because she realized she's the only one who can. "Before, when I didn't know who I was or what I wanted, I couldn't say no to anything,'' says Kelly, ''and people walked all over me. I had to recognize what *I* felt comfortable doing, and speak up about it. That's something I've been working on a lot in the last couple of years. If someone makes a demand on me that I feel is overstepping their bounds and inappropriate, I've learned to speak up and say no. I'm not afraid that they won't like me anymore.''

Self-assertion has been a significant issue for Monica as well. ''My therapist gave me an exercise — something that *I* should do for myself — and it was asking people for things,'' Monica says. ''Like asking even, 'Could you pass me the butter?' *Asking*. Or, 'Could you do this or that for me?' And giving myself permission to take up more space, to fill out more space.''

Learning to be assertive — to stand up to bullies — has helped Monica feel tremendous personal power. ''You have to learn to stand up for yourself, because no one else will,'' she says. ''It *is* difficult to say no. But when you say no, you can sometimes notice that other people are respecting you much more because you did.''

Perhaps the most important payoff is that the recovering anorexic begins to respect herself a lot more. Continually giving in, meekly acquiescing to others' demands, makes any woman feel like a wimp, because she's giving her power away, letting other people run her life and make decisions for her. In short, she's letting other people control her and that just fuels her anger. Of course, society tells us that ''nice women'' don't *get* angry. So she represses her anger, making little mental notches whenever something or someone hurts her, instead of venting it right then and there. The internalized anger festers and builds, until it finally explodes in volcano-like rage. (Then the anorexic feels guilty, because that wasn't ''very nice'' either.) Asserting anger more constructively, without falling into the well-worn rut of old patterns, is a hard lesson to learn. Yet it's an intrinsic part of the recovery process.

''Self-assertion was a big issue for me and it still is,''says Leslie, ''but I've reached a point where I can assert myself. I just have to watch the way I do it. Because if I say to my family, 'I'm really upset; I'm just really angry,' that's threatening to them, so they shut off all communication. So I've had to learn to approach it in a different way. That's what I'm working on now — being more reflective with my anger. I tend to be passive-aggressive with my anger—'You hurt me, so now I'm going to say something to hurt *you!*' I'm working on dealing with my anger more constructively. That's my current goal.''

Helena is working through the myth that expressing her anger is "not nice," that she'll drive others away if she lets them know she's angry. "At times, I'm still afraid to express my anger," she admits. "I'm still very afraid that people will be angry with me. It's as if I think the whole world will collapse if people get angry with me. That's one of the reasons you want to be so kind and helpful, because you're so afraid that people will be angry if you're not. But it keeps you from expressing who you really are, and that's not good.''

Monica knows the danger of not venting her feelings. "Before, I never got angry. I just buried it," she says. "But it *is* difficult to begin expressing your anger because it goes against being nice all the time. It's really hard—it's scary to get angry, to show it. But it's good, too. It [the anger] needs to get out in some way; it needs to be expressed. Because if it doesn't, you just try by starving to numb it, to erase it in some way. And that doesn't work either.''

When recovering women stop trying to numb, erase or deny their feelings, it's scary because a slew of buried feelings come rushing to the surface. It's confusing, because they never *felt* anything before. They were numb to their feelings and now all of a sudden, they find themselves immersed in them, and don't know when it's going to stop.

"It's real confusing for me right now," says Robin, "because for the first time in my life, I'm feeling a need to be close to people. I'm feeling a sense of not having a lot of my needs met and feeling a lot of emptiness inside. So I'm feeling I *need* those connections, but it seems with my family specifically, I'm pushing them away. They're trying to be there for me now, but I have a lot of anger directed toward them, because they weren't there for me in that kind of way when I was growing up. And it's strange to me now, so foreign, to have them talk to me or be interested in what I'm doing, or to be around me. So I have a lot to work on in relation to them.''

Robin admits she still has many fears about relationships. "Right now, I'm in the middle of therapy with it all," she says. "I'm just starting to get in touch with what some of the fears are.

I'm starting to get away from the eating disorder, because the issue is *not* the food. I'm just coming from behind that and starting to identify exactly what it is."

Through it all, Robin has learned a valuable lesson. "I think the biggest thing my experience with anorexia taught me is that I have to be able to express myself to people," she remarks. "I have to be able to actually say [what I mean]—to recognize and express my needs to someone. I cannot expect someone to read my mind or read my behaviors, to automatically know what it is that I need or want from them. That recognition has been a key for me."

Through this recovery process, the anorexic slowly allows herself to unfold. She listens to her inner self and what *she* wants and needs. Recovery is not instantaneous; it's a process, so it takes time.

"Before, I was lying so very much to myself," says Monica. "I built up some ideal person. I didn't know who I was, so I just figured out some person who I thought, 'That would be good.' Some days I was a femme fatale. Some days I was this radical feminist. And some days I was a hippie. I was really confused. I didn't know shit about who I was."

Monica has learned to be comfortable with the "gray areas" in her life. "Now I feel that I accept that I don't know exactly who I am," she says. "I know that I am very split up, but it's okay to be that. It's okay that some days, I may dress a little bit like this, and other days, a little bit like that. I'm very aware of what I'm doing, but I don't feel panicked about not knowing everything. I *know* that I don't know everything. Before, I didn't know. I thought I knew everything and that everything was under control. Now I know it isn't. And it's okay."

A key concept to learn in recovery is that life cannot be controlled. No matter what one does in trying to have everything going like clockwork, completely under control, the proverbial wrench inevitably drops out of the sky and destroys "the best-laid plans." Recovery means moving away from the structure of having to have everything spelled out in black-and-white, and learning to live in the gray areas—with all of the uncertainties—as well as all of the freedom and options and choices. There's no quick way to get over anorexia nervosa. It's a process of self-discovery, self-expression, and self-care.

"When you're into your food and weight obsessions," Brenda remarks, "you think there *is* a secret, there *is* a quick fix. Then you learn there's not. It's just learning to care enough about yourself that you're not going to do this self-destructive thing anymore."

Brenda believes she became anorexic as she endeavored to cope with the intense stress and pressure she felt in her life because of her low self-esteem. "I think that's the biggest reason for it," she says. "I allowed myself to do this destructive thing to myself because of a lack of self-esteem. That's why I think so much of recovering is learning to accept yourself and care for yourself. Because eating disorders are very self-destructive, and if you *care* about yourself, you don't want to do that. If you truly care about your well-being, you don't want to abuse and hurt yourself."

One of the most valuable lessons Brenda has learned in recovery is to listen to her inner self, to pay attention to her thoughts and feelings. "The whole thing with my eating disorder has made me realize that in order to live a happy life, I have to live an inspected life," she says. "I can't go through life just letting things happen and not thinking about them. I need to look for the underlying issues of what it means to me. If something happens, I have to inspect it. I have to analyze my life. Because there are a lot of issues I've had to deal with that I tried not to through my eating disorder. I think I've gained self-awareness that I never would have had. I've learned a lot about myself. I still have more to learn, but if it had not been for my eating disorder, I don't think I would have even started."

With this new-found self-awareness comes the freedom to choose. The recovering anorexic realizes that she holds the key and has the freedom to do whatever she wants. Yet it is important to remember that freedom is intrinsically tied to responsibility. She is free to do whatever she chooses, but must learn to accept the consequences for her actions.

"I've learned that it's definitely self-inflicted," Jessica remarks, "and if you're going to get over it, you're the only one who's going to do that. It's totally a one-person job. You can have help along the way, but it's not going to get you through recovery unless *you* want to do it. It's a very destructive disease and I have no one to blame but myself. I've really destroyed my body with it. It's very life-threatening and very destructive — in a lot of ways — isolation, your health, the whole person in general. It ruins a person.''

Yet Jessica must be forgiving and gentle with herself. While part of the process involves confronting the choices she has made and taking responsibility for her actions, she would best revel in the positive choices she has made toward wellness and recovery and not get stuck in self-blame.

"Everybody has problems and no one has an easy time in life," Nikki remarks, "and we have to use what we've been given and try to go with that. Because constantly concentrating on what we don't want and don't have is useless. I try to relax and be happy — and I wish I could do that more! But my struggle with anorexia has taught me a lot about being open with people. People aren't going to go away if you open up to them; they're probably going to come closer." When you express yourself and your needs, others will appreciate your honesty and openness. They *do* come closer. And often, they teach you all sorts of things — not only about themselves, but about you.

"I always used to keep pretty much to myself," says Nancy, "so I didn't know a lot about other people, because I didn't have that much contact with them in an intimate way. I was always very distanced. But I learned that it was okay — that I was not as abnormal as I thought I was if I had certain thoughts or did certain things. Other people shared or did things that sometimes made them feel dumb, too. Or they would do something and think later, 'Why did I do that?' Or, 'Why did I say that?' I began to realize that it was all right, and that I didn't have to beat myself up about it — that other people do the same thing. I learned an awful lot about other people — and myself, too." We *all* make mistakes. Sometimes we do and say things we wish we could take back. But there's no need to punish ourselves. We've all heard so many times that nobody's perfect; we just have to *believe* it.

"I'm *learning* to accept the fact that I'm never going to be perfect," says Jill, "because there *is* no perfection. At one time, I thought, 'Well, Christ is perfect; I'm going to be perfect.' But we're all human. We can't be perfect in the body. We can only be perfect in spirit.''

Making mistakes can be wonderful (in retrospect, that is). As Jill says, we can *learn* from our mistakes and can *grow* from them if we let ourselves. Looking back, mistakes can even be a little amusing.

Leslie laughs when she remembers herself in the hospital, not even *trying* anything she couldn't do *perfectly*. "I refused to go to art therapy at first," she says with a smile. "I didn't like art. Art was one thing that I didn't 'achieve' at, and I didn't want to do anything that I couldn't do well. I used to be the type that if I couldn't do something, I wouldn't even attempt it. So I really fought that class. But I got through it. And we didn't have to *draw* pictures, we could just use colors to express our feelings on themes that the instructor gave us. And it turned out to be one of the biggest things to get in touch with the emptiness I felt. Taking that chance and trying something new taught me a lot about myself.''

Leslie learned that the world wouldn't crumble if she didn't do everything perfectly. She began to try new things — like a child would — and not be afraid of failure because there was no shame. There were no "shoulds." Leslie began to accept herself exactly as she is.

Yet even when a recovering anorexic accepts herself and makes positive changes in her life, all the situations that used to drive her to starve herself do not suddenly disappear. In fact, in many ways, the challenges move onward and upward, yet gradually she learns that successfully conquering these challenges makes her even stronger.

Nancy remembers a particular situation that challenged her coping skills. "This woman called to set up an appointment for me to go in and get my job back, and she sounded so businesslike, so efficient on the phone," says Nancy. "I remember I got off the phone and I was a nervous wreck. I didn't eat all that day and I got real funny about it. I kept feeling 'fat' all day. It just so happened that I had an appointment with my therapist the following day, so I told him about it. And he said, 'That very clearly shows a correlation.' Even though I kept telling myself, 'I am *not* fat,' and I *knew* I was not fat, I felt 'fat' all day. And it was obviously the anxiety arising around this woman's phone call.''

Slowly, Nancy began to realize that while she couldn't change the situation, she *could* change her reaction. The first step toward this empowering change was recognizing the link between her anxieties and her perceptions of being "fat." When she became more aware of this connection, she could stop herself from acting on impulse and starving herself. Unearthing these issues, however, can be frightening and overwhelming. It's tough to be caught in a flood of confused feelings and anxieties, but the recovering anorexic learns that she can *choose* her reaction. Slowly, she begins to cope with these stressors in different ways.

"I used to never feel anything," says Monica, "but now I *feel* anxiety. I feel lots of anxiety. I find it very hard to concentrate very often — every day — so I have to live with that. It's because the therapy and my progress have raised so many feelings. But now, I don't starve over them. I've learned to think, 'This passes.' I can lie down or just . . . I know I won't die from it. I don't have to starve over it, because I know, 'Okay, maybe it's hard now and I'm tempted to stop eating.' But in some way, I think I have learned to relax a little, to be more conscious of what is going on inside of me. And not get into a panic and just see red and not know anything. I think I'm more familiar with my feelings."

"A trick I've learned is to objectify things a little bit," says Yvette. "I just say, 'Well, you know, I can look at a situation in a negative way, or I can look at it as a positive. It's my choice.' That has helped me a lot — just realizing this little objective truth that it's up to me. I can shine the bright light on it. And I get a little Pollyannish sometimes, but it helps. It helps a lot. Because I think I *do* see how momentary we are. This is my moment, and it's your moment, too — why not make it good? I mean, life's so short, you might as well."

. Jill has also learned to work through the rough spots. "I used to not want to feel that I had to go through the hard times," Jill remarks. "I used to think that I could avoid them and then just deal with the good things in life. But part of recovery is realizing it's *how* you cope with the hard times, *how* you deal with them. You can make the good bad, or the bad good. It's up to you."

Recognizing her right to choose has given Jill a stronger sense of her personal power. "I'm in control," she says, "but in control in the sense of how I cope with something. I'm obviously not in control with the food. I'm not in control with the physical, the exercise. But I *am* in control of how I feel about them. Maybe that's the only thing I'll ever learn to feel in control of."

The hard times and the challenges aren't going to go away. They'll still be there, even when anorexia nervosa has been overcome. As Chiara says, the key is learning to let go of ridiculous, perfectionistic demands. "I used to make these long lists," she says, "and if I didn't get through all of that stuff every day, I'd really feel like a failure. Part of my recovery was learning that there *is* a tomorrow. Because I always thought that I had to get everything done today."

The world won't come to an end if Chiara realizes that she doesn't get around to everything today. So much of it can be put off until tomorrow. Like many recovered anorexics, Chiara realizes the importance of relaxing a little, relaxing *a lot*, and taking good care of herself—because she's the only one who can. Now she makes choices that are *good* for her, and in her best interests—like getting enough sleep at night and exercising (regularly, but not obsessively).

Helena has also learned to strike that balance. "I like to exercise, but if I'm stressed and I want to exercise, it's different than it used to be," she says. "Before, if I wanted to go exercising, it was out of anxiousness. It was not relaxing; it just made me worse. I think it's good to exercise, because the body needs to exercise, but *not* obsessively, and not perhaps in *that* moment when you are very stressed and anxious, like you're ready to run a marathon. For me, it's just walking with my dog. I do that a lot. And then I feel calm and relaxed."

Slowing down and cutting down on the number of tasks she takes on is an important lesson for the recovering anorexic to learn. She doesn't have to do it all, be it all, have it all, but rather, take the time to play and have fun!

Brenda's form of play and fun is taking dance lessons again. "I took dance lessons the whole time I was growing up," she says. "It was a lot of fun for me and I really missed it. So I started up again about a year ago. I take dance lessons three times a week. And you know, it's odd because when I was anorexic, I exercised every day.

But that was because I had this fear that I would be fat if I didn't. Now I do this because I really enjoy it."

Chiara has also learned to take the pressure off of herself, to goof around, play, and have fun. "I've had to learn to do other things," she says. "I've gotten more involved with my friends and with dancing. I *love* to dance. Almost every month, I'm trying to get my friends to go dancing. I love to just *be* with my friends."

Other women rekindle their passions for music and art — for going to concerts and movies and museums, to get away from it all. Some try sports they never dared, like tennis, golf, or horseback riding. Others try reading fiction for the first time — all the classics they never had time for — but, steer clear of those anxiety-provoking women's magazines!

Helena has learned other ways of taking a break from the stress — shutting it all off, when it gets to be too much. "Today, when I feel lots of stress and many demands, it's because I'm wanting to do my best — too much — and so I get very tired," Helena says. "But I've learned to shut it off. I go for walks or meet my friends or call them on the phone and talk. I do something that *I* want to do. I've learned to slow down and have a moment for myself."

Talking with friends is a key coping strategy for Helena now. "I understand my feelings the most after talking with my friends," she says. "Even though they didn't have this experience with anorexia, just talking to other people — just to *tell* them, to have someone else listen — that helps the pressure and demands go away. Because I feel they love me and accept me, no matter what."

Helena first learned how to let go of pressures and demands while on holiday in Spain. It was a new experience for her, and it changed her life forever. "At first, I thought, 'No, I don't want to go to Spain because I have many things to do,'" Helena remembers, "and I did not think it was a good idea. But finally, I ended up going to Spain with a friend whose parents had a house there. And it was a really good week, because there was no stress and no demands. I had a lot of time to think about what I wanted to do. But I also had time to leave myself — to look out to what's happening outside, to just be in the moment, just now. What's happening here just now."

Helena learned to live in the present, and not get hung up on pressures and anxieties about the future. She learned to appreciate the moment and *be* in it. "Sometimes you have to lose your head, to lose all sense of space and time, to just be here and now," Helena says. "I learned it that week in Spain and it was very good. But then I came back to Sweden, and I had much to do at work. But then I started to remind myself, 'I have to just be in the moment. So what will I do? How can I do the best thing? I have to just be in the moment.' And that is the way I cope with stress today."

A recovering anorexic has to learn to maximize her choices in the moment. It's a strategy with tremendous power. If the issues seem too confusing and too overwhelming, she needs to let go of them, even if it's just for a little while, and make the best choices right now. Granted, there will be slip-ups. A recovering anorexic's old way-of-coping is so ingrained and such a part of her past that it may seem instinctual. It may be her gut-level first response, but she realizes the need to seize the opportunity, move on to the next step and think of alternatives to make the best choice in the moment. Falling into old patterns happens at times . . . maybe a lot at first . . . and then less and less often. The recovering anorexic learns to forgive herself, to be gentle and kind with herself. She begins to appreciate what's happening just now—and savor the moment.

Chapter 8

Meaning

When a woman is in the throes of a struggle with anorexia nervosa, she can't imagine what life would be like without endlessly obsessing about thinness, weight, and calories. What else could she possibly focus on? What could she think about? What would she do? What would she be?

Once mired in these obsessions, Helena clung to them desperately. She didn't think she could ever live without them. Or would ever want to. As Helena remembers, "The doctor told me, 'The day will come when you can leave all these thoughts about food and being thin or fat, and then it will be no problem for you.' And I thought, 'How can I ever, ever, leave these thoughts?' But I *can*, I think," says Helena. "And perhaps, in a little bit of time, I will leave them forever."

Before an anorexic can stop these obsessive thoughts, her weight must stabilize and, of course, this doesn't happen overnight. Often, there are issues holding her back. Chiara is starting to understand why maintaining her weight is so scary. "I've come to realize why every time I'm at the weight I am now, I can't stand it—I can't tolerate it because I feel like my mother," she says. "When I look into the mirror, I don't see me—I see my mother. When I'm at a more normal weight, I can't tolerate that. That's why I'm having difficulty right now staying where I'm at because to me, I feel like my mother—that I am a part of her—and I have to separate from that. I kind of lose my identity when I get to be a normal weight."

At least now, Chiara is aware of the issues. And that's a solid step forward. "I've gained so much insight working on the issues in the last two years," she says, "that even though it's still a struggle,

I have a hold on it. I know my signals now, so I'm more aware of that. I'm able to express more to my therapist."

Chiara is able to eat regular, balanced meals, but it wasn't always like that. "When I was at my worst, I would tell myself that no matter how much or how little I ate, it wouldn't fill the emptiness I felt inside," she says. "Or numb it. Sometimes, when I was really sick, I'd go out and watch people eat — and I'd cry, because I'd say, 'Why can't *I* do that? Why is it so hard?' And it's still a struggle. But I've learned to get up and dust myself off and say, 'Yesterday was a bad day. Let's start all over again.' Whereas before, I would say, 'The hell with this,' and just keep going down."

The real key, Chiara has found, is changing her behavior. The same feelings, the same issues will come up, but as she works through recovery, she learns to deal with them more constructively.

For the first time in her life, Robin realizes that she is too thin and her weight needs to be higher. "Throughout the time that I was in the hospital, I was never happy with my weight and my image of myself was always distorted," she says. "But now, I'm *trying* to eat a lot more and *trying* to gain."

Robin needed to work through other issues before she could handle gaining weight. "When I started losing so much weight, everybody just wanted to talk about eating and weight," she remarks, "and I kept trying to say to them that there are so many issues going on in my life out there in the world, and that's what we needed to focus on more. That's what I've found in my recovery. The more I work on the relationship issues and things like that, the easier it is for me to eat."

For Alison, the issue is the symbolism of weight. "It's difficult because I was heavy as a child and it's something I've vowed that will never happen again," she says, "so I think keeping it gradual is helping."

Alison had been maintaining her weight for some time when we spoke. "It was just kind of touch and go when I was discharged from the hospital," she admits. "I left before I even got a chance to finish the program because my insurance ran out. I've had to do a lot of struggling on my own since I left the hospital, so for *me* to maintain, it's pretty good."

Alison doesn't even own a scale anymore. "I get weighed at my doctor's once a week, and I don't even look," she says. "I turn my back, so I don't know what it is. He'll tell me whether I'm up or down, but he won't tell me from what point, and I find that very helpful."

Because Alison feels she needs help in planning her meals, she sees a nutritionist once a month and follows a food exchange list — eating a certain number of fruit and vegetable, protein, dairy, and bread exchanges each day. "I think it works well because it doesn't allow me to obsess about things," Alison says. "Because if I know I'm going to have this at this time, I don't have to worry — 'Oh my God, do I need to starve all day so I can eat dinner?' It's a program that's there, so it doesn't allow me to obsess."

Slowly, Alison says she's *starting* to see herself more accurately. "It goes back and forth," she admits. "Sometimes I'll look and see exactly what I look like, and sometimes I won't. I think it has to do with how much stress I've been under or how I'm feeling. If I'm upset, I'm more inclined to see myself as heavier."

Like all women in recovery, Alison sometimes experiences slip-ups and setbacks. "Occasionally, I'll do things like look through the exchange list and find what's the lowest calories," she says with a grin. "Or I'll think that I've binged — after eating four crack-ers or something — and not eat the next meal. But that's happening less and less."

Most significantly, Alison *copes* differently after eating what she perceives to be a binge. "The most important thing has been just changing my thinking," she says. "Before, I used to think, 'Well, I've blown it once, why don't I just keep screwing up? If I eat a cracker, forget it, I may as well eat the whole pack.' I think I've changed it to, 'Well okay, I made a mistake, I just need to get right back to it.' That's how I handle it now."

At times, Alison is tempted to cope "the old way," but that's natural. Starving over feelings and anxieties is such an ingrained way-of-coping. The change now is, she handles it differently. She doesn't see it as right or wrong, good or evil. She acknowledges that she made a mistake (with no blame or guilt!), picks herself up, and keeps going.

Recovery is a gradual process. A woman can't expect to wake up one day and quit anorexia nervosa "cold turkey." It's not the same as giving up coffee or cigarettes, because food is needed to survive. Consequently, there are many tests every day. But in time, recovering women learn to make the "right" choices, in their own best interests, more and more often.

"There have been times when I've been *tempted* to just take one or two laxatives," Nancy admits, "but I don't even have any in the house. And there have been times when I've maybe eaten too much bran or something to deliberately induce diarrhea if I'm afraid I'm starting to get too heavy. But most of the time, I'm able to keep things pretty well on an even keel. I know I've got a lot to lose if I slip back into it — and not just weight."

Nancy doesn't have an *intense* desire to lose weight anymore. "I wanted to [lose weight] *desperately* before. When I lost a half a pound, I'd have to lose another tomorrow," she says. "Sometimes, though, I still feel like I don't want to go up beyond a certain weight, so I feel if I lose a little, that provides me with a little safety margin. But at the same time, I know if I do that, if I lose *too* much, then I get myself in real trouble."

Nancy is making a conscious effort to eat more, more often. "I *still* eat a lot of low calorie things," she admits, "but a lot of times, I *will* go ahead and drink a can of Ensure (a meal-in-a-can supplement) rather than eating, if for some reason, I decide I don't want to eat or I'm in a hurry and know that I *should* eat. Like if I'm on my way to work and I don't have time, then I will go ahead and drink a can of Ensure. Even though I know it's 250 calories. The bigger can is 365 calories. But I still will go ahead and drink that. *That*, I think, has made a big difference. Before, I wouldn't bother with anything."

Nancy feels she's functioning better than she used to. "I notice now a big difference in the way that I'm performing at work compared to the way I was performing when I was at 70 or 72," she says. "There *is* a big difference, and a lot of it has to do with concentration and energy. Before, I had lots of energy, but it was very nervous energy — very hyper. I couldn't sit still. I was jumping around, running around, and that's when I was using laxatives. I was also using diuretics, so I was spending a lot of time in the bathroom, too. And you can't really be helping the public if you're in the bathroom," Nancy laughs.

When a recovering anorexic truly cares about her well-being, she acts in her own best interests. As a friend of mine often reminds me, "Behavior doesn't lie." That's why, even if a recovering anorexic doesn't like it sometimes, she *makes* herself eat.

"I *try* to eat three meals a day," Deborah remarks, "but eating is still not my favorite thing to do. I don't enjoy it. It's not pleasurable for me, but I know I have to do it. So I make myself eat."

Slowly, recovering women learn to make more positive choices — for themselves, instead of against themselves. Eventually they break out of their denial and admit that yes, they *do* need food to survive, just like everyone else.

For Helena, this is the real key: simply eating to live. "I think if you can leave all the thoughts about thinness and talks about dieting, then it will *be* no problem," Helena remarks. "You can eat what you want to. Sometimes, you can even eat something that is not so good for you."

"It's not easy, I know," Helena says, "but it would be so much better if you could just concentrate on doing all the things in your life first. And then if you are on 'E,' [empty] like a car that has to have some petrol, you eat exactly what you need."

Helena is listening to her body — paying attention to the hunger cues, instead of ignoring them, and eating in response to these signals. When she does this, maintaining her weight is easy. It's a simple concept. All it takes is eating exactly what she needs, exactly what she's craving, and stopping when she has had enough. As Susie Orbach (1978) advocates, it's a matter of eating in response to "stomach hunger," rather than "mouth hunger."[1] In other words, when one *feels* hungry, one *eats* (instead of ignoring it!) — and eats enough to satisfy the hunger.

I strongly believe that anorexics cannot set up food to be "the enemy" in recovery, because they are only setting themselves up to fail. I feel it's very important not to make any foods taboo or off-limits. Anorexics have spent so much time doing that; as they recover, it's time to give themselves the freedom to make choices.

In time, recovering women learn to strike their own balances.

They discover what works best for them. When they follow their own inner guidance and eat in response to their hunger cues, maintaining their weight isn't a problem.

Brenda's golden rule is eating three meals a day. "I used to skip breakfast, but I think breakfast is very important," she says. "I like meat, but I don't like to fix it, so I don't fix it. I'll eat it in a restaurant. At lunch, I'll have yogurt—I mix up yogurt and a banana and granola. And people think that [because of] what I'm eating, I'm *dieting*. But I eat that because I *like* it.

"I have become very aware of trying to eat healthy foods," adds Brenda. "I don't like to eat a lot of processed foods. I don't eat at McDonald's and places like that because I don't care for it. I guess it's basically just a matter of finding what you like to eat and then eating it. And I try not to eat so that I feel really stuffed, especially my evening meal, because I don't like to go to bed feeling really full. But I haven't made any foods taboo—because I think that just sets you up."

This is where Brenda's philosophy departs from Overeaters Anonymous. "To me, never being able to eat sugar again—it's not normal," Brenda says. "I'll get dessert in a restaurant, or if I'm having dinner at someone's house, I'll have dessert, but I don't feel crazy about it and think that, 'Oh my God, I better not eat for the next three days because I ate this and I'm so bad.' And it's not like I've never overeaten since I've been recovering. But I think that's normal, too. Normal people will sit down and eat a huge meal every once in a while. The thing is, when I finish, I finish. Before, it would be, 'Well, I've blown the whole day, let's just continue eating the rest of the day.'"

When Brenda first started recovering, she says she had to learn how to deal with food in a "normal" way again. "When I started eating three meals a day again, I thought that I was eating too much," she says. "I thought, 'How can I eat this much? I'm going to get fat!' But I didn't."

After a while, Brenda realized she could throw away her scale. Once she began listening to her body and eating in response to it, she didn't need the scale for security anymore because her weight was no longer an issue.

Joanna agrees. "Food and eating are really on the fringes of my life, she says." "The only things I don't eat are octopus and bananas. I eat *everything*. Sometimes, though, I'll drink a diet Coke just because I don't want the heavy sugar in a Coke, but a lot of times I'll make myself drink the sugared version because I need the calories. I *do* think about needing the calories, because I'm still on the thin side, and if I get into a real stressful time, I tend to lose my appetite."

Joanna tries to get a reasonable – but not obsessive – amount of exercise. "I work downtown and walk to work," she says, "and my husband and I are avid bicyclists. There's a pool nearby, although I can't say I swim I lot. But I think just biking on the weekend – that's enough. I really *do* eat – I'll slather the butter on my baked potato. I'm so aberrant now, I eat the way I like to. But I listen to my body now and eat what I want and need."

Once recovering women begin feeling comfortable with their weight and comfortable with themselves, they look around and see the societal preoccupation with thinness and appearance with new insight.

In most Western societies, women have been socialized to define themselves – to express their identities – through appearances. For ages the realm of appearances has been thrust upon women as the key to success. In today's world, women are encouraged to be "Superwomen" and excel in careers, too – but still do *not* receive equal pay for equal work, nor equal power and respect, nor even equal opportunities. Infuriatingly enough, the beauty ideals are still around. Women are *still* encouraged to define themselves through their appearances. With beauty ideals changing as quickly as a season's new fashions, it's no surprise that there are still many women whose lives revolve around relentlessly trying to "perfect the shell." Women have been socialized to act this way.

This realization hit home with Joanna. "One thing became self-evident to me the other day with a receptionist at work," Joanna remarks. "She's terribly vain, and she has a little mirror that no one can see but her, and she's constantly there. We had this discussion – well, she'd had her eyes done about ten years ago and I was curious about it. Well, she was getting really emotional about it, and all of a sudden, it became very clear to me that the very essence of the way she sees herself and judges herself as being an 'okay' person is whether she's physically beautiful. She must not like herself at all on the inside because it consumes her. That was sort of an exaggerated example to me that when your outside becomes so important, then you must not like what's on the inside.''

Society cultivates this ideal in women—to not concern oneself with inner qualities, but be totally fixated on appearances. When many women don't meet ever-changing beauty ideals—as no one can, no matter how great the gene pool—they hate themselves.

Perhaps there's a stronger societal motive in keeping women eternally preoccupied with "perfecting the shell." In addition to racking up profits for the beauty and fashion industries, "perfecting the shell" takes up so much of a woman's time and energy that there's nothing left to direct anywhere else. It keeps women out of potentially threatening arenas like politics, policy issues, and upper management, where women could make a powerful difference. It prevents women from participating in the world on an equal basis, and it works so well!

As the anorexic recovers, she finds that it's not easy to stand up and revolt against societal pressures. So many people just don't see the marked preoccupation with thinness as a feminine ideal. Or perhaps, they just don't want to listen. The fixation on women's appearances is so ingrained in society, many don't know any other way-of-being.

This infuriates Joanna. "I want to shake people up and tell them that there's so much more to life than what you look like," she says. "But the whole thinness obsession is really overdone in the media. And because I'm naturally thin, it bothers me the way other women respond to me. 'Oh you're so lucky to be that thin!' I think, 'Well, you know, it's terribly superficial to only look at the physical aspect of a person, because I think of everybody as having so much more to them.' But that's the message that's driven home in our society," Joanna remarks. "When I go home and visit with all of my high school friends, they'll talk about their kids and their weight. I mean, that's a real focus point for them, the condition of their weight. I'm just interested in so many other things right now that I'm not *thinking* about my weight. I remember the last time I went to visit a friend, it was a big issue to her that I didn't notice her weight loss. And I was thinking to myself, 'Well I didn't come to see how much weight she lost. I came to see *her.*'"

Trying to fight the intense societal pressure is extremely frustrating. "It seems in our society, most people can only base their judgments of other people on the outside," Joanna observes. "It's very superficial, but it's most common. But I'm interested in the *person.* The *whole person.*"

With so much emphasis placed on a woman's appearance, Brenda says its not surprising that most of the women she knows are extremely uncomfortable with their bodies. "The women I know just seem to be really screwed up about their bodies—even 'normal' women," Brenda says. "There's this one woman I work with and she's shorter than I am, and she's pretty solid—muscular—but she's not fat at all. And she's always saying that she has such huge hips and that she's really fat in that area. Well, I went to the beach one time with a group of women from work, and she had on a bathing suit and she's tiny! She's small. And I thought, 'Here's a woman, she doesn't have an eating disorder, she's so-called "normal," and she's pretty much obsessed with how her body is, that she's fat in that area.'"

The obsession with extreme thinness hit Brenda with quite a jolt when she looked back on her anorexic days. "When I was at my lowest weight, I was getting a lot of compliments from other women and a lot of attention from men," Brenda remarks. "And you know, when I think about it, getting that attention is really kind of sick. The other thing is, my parents never said . . . it was like they were never alarmed that I was so thin. And I think that's pretty sick, too. That's what makes me so angry—that extreme thinness is so worshipped and coveted in our society—that you're unhealthy and people think it's great. I *know* I really looked sick, because I *was* really sick."

Consequently, Brenda has placed a great deal of emphasis on trying to ignore societal pressures in her recovery. "It's just learning to accept my body as I am," she says. "I know one thing I used to do was put off my life, waiting to lose that next five pounds. You know, 'When I lose five pounds, then a man will be attracted to me.' And now, it's just learning to live today. 'Well, this is my body today. This is what I have to work with today.' So I don't want to wait to lose the five pounds."

When recovering women start to accept themselves as they are, they can take a stand against societal pressures. It doesn't matter what society says, the only thing that matters is that she's happy. And maybe, just maybe, she can be an example for others.

In *Women & Self-Esteem*, Linda Tschirhart Sanford and Mary Ellen Donovan (1985) point out that a woman has the power to choose. She can refuse to go along with ideals that are oppressive, and not her own. She can take control by expressing her personal power—by refusing to judge herself against such defeating ideals, refusing to support the plethora of beauty industries that only serve to keep women down, and speaking up when she sees or hears advertising that bothers her.[2]

"I've learned not to listen to what society says, because society isn't always right," Kelly remarks. "I refuse to read *Cosmo* or any of those magazines that only try to destroy your self-esteem. I *love* who I am now—and I will never, ever try to change myself to conform to someone else's ideal again!"

Gradually, a woman's perspective on weight changes. "I've kind of gone overboard the other way," Leslie says with a laugh. "If I look at a model or something, I'll say, 'She's starved, she's starved.' They kind of ingrained that in the hospital—that so many of the models you see are anorexic. And when you see someone like that, you realize you don't want to be like them. You think, 'Oh, no, no, no—that starved person must be unhappy.'"

Heidi doesn't want to be *thin*; she just wants to be healthy. "My taste has changed," Heidi says. "I don't like *thin* anymore. I like healthy. That's my reaction to the society thing, the media thing—because it's *unhealthy*. Now I look at models and just say, strictly from an aesthetic point of view, 'She's too thin.' It's not bitterness. It's not envy. It's just an aesthetic."

Heidi has taken a stand against this societal fixation. She refuses to get involved in anything that supports the appearance obsession. "I refuse to get involved in diet talk or workout talk with friends. I just refuse to go along with it," Heidi says. "It makes me very angry. It really does."

Helena observes that the women she knows who are obsessed

with dieting are mainly those who don't need to diet. "Where I work now, they sometimes talk about dieting, and I never want to be involved in a discussion about dieting or anything like that. By now, I have been through so many phases of this, I don't want to listen to it. I've realized it's not important. I get sad when people talk about dieting," Helena adds, "because there's so much more in life. There are so many more important things. And it makes me feel sad because I knew there was a time in my life when that was the most important thing. But at that time, I didn't know there was anything else."

Helena has a chilling recollection of when she began dieting. "When I started to get anorexia, at least one or two women said to me, 'You're quite lucky because you are starting so early.' It makes me sad when I think about it." Yet in retrospect, Helena says maybe she *did* start early. "With all the things I have been through, I have grown a lot," Helena says. "It's really sad when I think that many women spend their whole lives concerned with food and weight and thinness. I know that I am much more grown [mature] than many women in their 30s or 40s. And now, for the first time in my life, I can say that I'm truly happy."

For Heidi, the real changes and growth toward happiness occurred after she began moving outside of herself and her narrow concerns with calories and thinness. "One of the most important turning points in my recovery was a wonderful surprise when I was putting on weight and people were complimenting me, and complimenting me on my personality change," Heidi says. "Then I started to realize what was so important, what was the attraction. After I gained weight, I started appreciating other people and appreciating myself and that's when I started feeling okay, really okay with myself. I started realizing that other things are more important than what you look like. Other people could be genuinely interested in you, and I just became a lot happier with everything else in my life. It had been so long since I had a very close friendship with anybody, and when I was 19 or 20, I suddenly had two very, very strong girlfriends."

The real key for Heidi was learning to be less selfish. "When I look at anorexia now, I think it's such a selfish, selfish disease," Heidi says. "I want to shake people up and say, 'What's the matter with you?! Don't you see what you're doing to other people and yourself, and what you're missing out on?' I think it's so stupid.''

The difference now, is that Heidi has learned to appreciate the inner qualities of a person more than anything. "Your personality and how you feel about yourself and other people are so much more important than what you look like," Heidi remarks. "And if people are going to put a premium on just an outer appearance, then don't worry about them, don't deal with them. I don't worry about other people's opinions as much anymore. I just go on being what I am, rather than what I think other people think I should be.''

Throughout an anorexic's recovery, when she starts to see clear differences between the person she was and the person she has become, she finds the shift in how she perceives others startling. "I've started looking at people as people, instead of what they look like," Alison remarks. "I think I've gone from being different from other people because I felt so inferior or ugly or so fat or whatever, to feeling different because I see positive things. But it's not like I'm unacceptably different . . . just different.''

In time, as recovering women gain self-acceptance, they realize their power in expressing needs and desires. "I have a lot more assertiveness now," remarks Joanna. "I have a lot more feeling that I have a right to pursue my interests, in that I really feel that I'm an important person. I understand more what kind of a person I am, and I accept parts of myself that before I didn't — the fact that I'm more of an introverted type, as opposed to the 'party animal' sort of character. It still bothers me a little bit, that I'm not at ease in all kinds of situations. But I certainly have come a long way.''

Joanna *accepts* that she's not perfect now, and doesn't have to be. Gradually, recovering women start to realize that they don't *have* to measure up to some ideal standard. All they need to do is be themselves and the rest will start to unfold.

"I have hated myself a lot in the past," Helena remarks, "but I think that changed as I started to find myself, to do things on my own. When I started my education, for example — it wasn't easy always — but again, I was trying to be my own person. That *means* something. You have to start getting to know who you are and do something that you like, so you can feel, 'That's me,'" Helena adds. "For me, when I finished my education, then I thought, this is *my* life. This is me."

Slowly, recovering women start discovering what they want to *do* with their lives. Abraham Maslow (1971) uses the term "self-actualization" to describe the process of finding something you believe in—discovering your calling, purpose, your mission that seems to fit who you are like a key in a lock.[3] Granted, sometimes it means backtracking a little. As Brenda began recovering, she realized that the profession she chose in college was the safe and secure option, but it wasn't what she *really* wanted to do.

"It's funny because I majored in business, and I knew going into my freshman year that that's what I was going to major in," Brenda remarks. "But when I took my business courses, I really didn't *like* them. I'm working in business now, but I have never really *liked* it. I think I chose it because it's very controlled, very safe, you can make a comfortable living at it. But now, I'm exploring a career change—something that would suit me much better—like human resource management."

Chiara's "true calling" has emerged through her recovery as well. When she was anorexic, she couldn't see a future for herself. "I felt empty all my life, until recently," says Chiara. "I felt like I was just existing. I could never see myself in the future. I could never see what value I would have in the future. I felt I was just acting, playing a role for someone else."

Back then, going to school and pursuing something she loved was just a dream for Chiara. "But now I'm doing something concrete to make it a reality," Chiara says. "It gives me hope that I *can* accomplish all of my dreams. And looking at the progress I've made tells me there is a future. I *know* there is something waiting for me."

In recovery, an anorexic must dare to follow her heart—no matter what anyone else says. Even if whatever she wants to do seems a little impractical or far-fetched to others, she owes it to herself to at least try—to give it a shot, whether it's a professional goal, or just for fun. After all, what has she got to lose?

Helena has gotten back in touch with a true passion that she left behind many years ago—singing. "I'm not sure what I will do with it," Helena says. "For the moment, I *do* think it's good to be where

I work. But I love to sing. And when I was sick, some years went by that I didn't sing at all. But now that I have started to sing a little bit, I've realized that just in the last year—when I've been feeling better—I found that I could sing better. So now I have these thoughts that maybe I should take a little break from work and just see what I can do with the singing. I don't think I want to make a living as a singer, but I like it very much. I can sit at the piano and the hours just go by. I lose myself in what I am doing and I don't think about food or eating, because music makes me so happy."

That's precisely what is looked for in recovery—something that is enjoyed so much that one gets lost in it. Whether it's a hobby, or simply play, it's taking time out to pursue the things that are enjoyed. That's what finding true passion is all about.

Monica's art is her passion. "It's happiness, pure happiness," Monica says. "That's what I think life is really all about—finding something that you can lose yourself in. Then eating and dieting and weight seem so unimportant. Because you realize those obsessions are *stopping* you from doing what you love. You realize you have something to be *well* for, to be able to do the things that you want to do. And I think that my painting, combined with people— because I now realize that people are very important to me, to feel that other people *need* me and I need them—that's very important. And that's *part* of my art. I think for me, painting is first, because time stops and everything," Monica adds. "Then you see you have this purpose. You show your work in exhibitions to people, you get their reactions and people recognize themselves or start to think in some new ways. Then you feel it's so meaningful."

Recovering women wonder how they ever lived with anorexia— so caught up in obsessions with food, weight and thinness when they had so many other gifts to offer. If only they could have understood, back then, how rich and full their lives could be. If only they could have understood what it was like to feel that their lives had "meaning."

Viktor Frankl, a psychologist whose theories are rooted in his experiences of surviving four concentration camps during the Holocaust, believes there are three ways to find meaning in life: (1) creating a work or deed that is authentically "you"; (2) loving another person; or, (3) when confronted by a situation one cannot change, transforming a tragedy into a personal triumph. "When we are no longer able to change a situation," Frankl writes, "we are challenged to change ourselves."[4]

The recovering anorexic does have the power to change – to transform the pain and suffering that once cut so deeply into personal triumph. As Chiara illustrates, she can't erase her experience with anorexia nervosa, but she *can* grow and change. She can become a much stronger person.

"I wouldn't wish this on my worst enemy," Chiara remarks. "Yet it *has* made me a stronger person. I don't know if I would have had the same insight that I have now if I didn't have something that was so life-threatening that it forced me to look at things."

Years later, when recovered women look back on their struggles with anorexia nervosa, they see it in a much different light. They realize how much they've grown since that time and how many positive coping skills they've gained. They're more secure with themselves and they cope differently. For instance, Chiara can accept criticism more constructively. She's not quite as sensitive as she was. "I'm learning that when someone says something to me, it doesn't mean the entire *person* is bad," Chiara says. "It just means that they're saying, 'Hey Chiara, do you realize you're doing this? You might want to look at it.' It's not an attack on all of me."

Recovering women learn not to blame *themselves* when they feel that others are reacting negatively to them. They don't live to please other people anymore. "If other people are reacting badly, maybe it's because of stress going on in their lives," Helena remarks. "If the way people are reacting to me is not good, it may be because of their thoughts. They may be having a bad day, or maybe situations in their lives are not going so well. But that's not *my* fault. I have also learned that. And you have to accept that not all people can understand you, because not everyone communicates in the same way."

Alison has also learned not to personalize criticism. "I've learned that there are just going to be people in the world who don't like you," Alison says. "Not everybody likes everybody, and I've learned to realize that it isn't necessarily *me*. It's just that this person and I just don't match."

As recovering women feel more secure in their own identities, they accept themselves as they are, with no excuses. This is when their relationships with others begin to change.

Since Alison began her recovery, her relationship with her parents has gotten much stronger. "I think it's better because I'm different," Alison says. "For a long time, I kind of held in my head that if *they* would change, then I would get better. But I'm starting to realize that they are how they are. They're not going to change and I can't do anything to change them. I just need to learn how to live my life with them being how they are."

Not getting "hooked" into the same behavior patterns is still a challenge, though. "My dad will size me up when he first sees me," Alison laughs, "and he won't say anything the whole time I'm there unless I'm getting ready to leave. Then he'll just bombard me with what he thinks. It's like I'm playing a game, but I've learned to *expect* this, so it doesn't bother me."

Sometimes separating geographically from family is needed, to give recovering women the space to explore and express their identities. Chiara explains, "I've been here for almost three years, and I don't have any desire to go back home now. *This* is home now. It was very important for me to separate from that family environment to start working on myself and my identity. I stay in touch with them," Chiara adds, "but the confusion is that they're not the same people that they were before, just as I'm not the same person I was before. My mother is happier now, because she's married and she has a new life. Her life has settled down a lot more and she's not the same person I remember. My sisters are different, my relatives are different, and it's confusing to me, because I still have all this anger and this bitterness, and where am I going to put it all?! I've found that family therapy has helped a little with that. And also realizing that they're never going to be the family that I wanted. I know I have to find the nurturing and support I need through other means."

The lesson for Helena in building her relationship with her mother has been to be "in the present," and not get hung up on the past. "Sometimes when I'm with my mother, she'll say something and I'll get so frustrated," says Helena, "but it's not because of what she's saying now. It's all the things she said ten or fifteen years ago—and they're still in my head."

Helena has learned to listen to what her mother is saying *now*, and shut the rest of it out. "Now my relationship with my mother is good," Helena says. "There are difficult times, but I can cope with them better. And I think if you take the time, you can understand why things were the way they were. I didn't have a bad childhood, but my mother was a dancer and a choreographer [and was disabled]. Today, her mind and her thoughts are very good—she is not depressed—but 15 years ago, 10 years ago, she was very depressed. I understand that now. Like I said before, sometimes you meet people and it's not so good and it could be that they're not feeling well, and that's what it was. She wasn't feeling well."

Helena believes it's very important not to get stuck in the past, and not to blame anorexia on parents or a difficult childhood. "Some women did, of course, have a difficult childhood, but others don't make any effort to understand what was happening at the time," Helena remarks. "Once you try to understand, you can move beyond it—to concentrate on what is happening just now—and forget all the rest. Some women just talk about their bad childhood or something and that just gets stuck in their thoughts. They keep going over it again and again and again and never move out of it. But the important thing is to leave it and just get in the moment. If you can't pull away from your angry or sad or frustrated memories, they ruin the moment. So you have to be . . . listening and hearing and thinking *now*, and try to forget bad memories and things."

Helena believes that "being in the moment" is important in every aspect of her life. "Sometimes, it's just the little things," she says with a laugh. "Sometimes small things, if you want to do them, you should. I remember last week, I was going to the subway, and there weren't many people. The stairs were nearly empty, but I thought, 'I don't want to go straight down, I want to go like this [zigzag].' You have to do what you want to do. If you want to go zigzag, you go zigzag. An important part of recovery is being your own person, laughing and being playful and sometimes a little bit crazy."

Brenda has learned not to wait around for others to make her happy, but to do things for herself, that make *her* happy. "One of the big turning points for me was the first fall after I started recovering," Brenda remarks. "I bought myself a strand of pearls. I had always wanted one, and you know, usually with expensive jewelry, you think, 'Well, a man is supposed to buy me that.' That was the first sign that I was starting to believe that I was worthy of something like that."

Brenda has changed in another way: She doesn't feel she "needs a man" to make her life complete. "I'm not seeing anyone now and I feel real good about it," Brenda says. "Before, it was like I *had* to have a man—if I didn't, I felt really worthless. But now, when someone is treating me badly, I'm not going to stand for it. Earlier this year, I was dating a guy for about three months, and he was very insensitive and I think that he's probably going to become an alcoholic. He drank just about every day, and would get drunk just about every time he drank. He eventually moved away, but I was starting to think, 'Wait a minute. I deserve a lot better than this.' And once he moved away, I called him up and said, 'I just think it would be better if we didn't talk to each other for a while.' An issue that I've been dealing with is that you learn a certain way of behaving back when you're anorexic and you're not healthy. And then you become healthier, but since this is the behavior you know, changing the behavior is a lot harder. It takes time. Yes, I initially attracted him, but then I knew that he was not a good person for me. Since I've been recovering, I feel I have a lot more choice in the matter. Before, I just felt so fortunate that someone would think that I was attractive enough to ask me out that I would leap at the chance."

The changes Brenda has seen in herself are remarkable. "I feel so much better about myself now than I did then," Brenda remarks. "I look way better now, and I think it's because I feel so much better about myself. My therapist said you can tell by the way that I walk, from when I first walked into her door. She says, 'It's like you're a totally different person.'"

When a recovered anorexic is happy with herself, she can reach out to others and not be so isolated anymore. "Now, when I am 25, my new life starts," Helena remarks. "As a teenager, when other people went out or met other people and had fun, I just sat in my room, studying my subjects for school or working by myself. I didn't want to meet other people. Sometimes I feel sad, because I spent so much of my life doing that. But I have many things to do now. Also, I gained so many experiences, I have no regrets. I wouldn't be the person I am today if I hadn't been through this.''

As the recovered anorexic looks back on what she has been through, she begins to comprehend the sheer magnitude of what she has experienced and the power she has to help others.

Monica now realizes she can make a difference. "My theory is, the only way you can help other anorexics is if you get involved in some organization," she says. "You have to talk to the women who come there."

Slowly, the recovered women begin to grasp that what they know, what they've been through, could save another woman's life. By sharing their insights and experiences, they could save another woman from going through what they did.

Helena, for example, volunteers as a resource person for her local anorexic organization. "Every day, we have one or two hours in which different people answer the telephone," Helena says. "So I do this one or two times a week—I answer the telephone. I didn't get involved in the organization until after I was recovered. I didn't want to be coming to them, searching for help. I wanted to be helping others. I felt better in November of last year, so in January, I contacted the anorexia organization and said, 'Now I want to get involved.' I wanted to stand on the square with other people—just shouting out—because it was ten or twelve years of my life. I can't just put them away. I think this is part of my recovery, to help other women. I *can* help other women.''

Once recovered, these women realize they *can* help other women because they understand, better than anyone, how a woman becomes anorexic. They recognize that society teaches women to define themselves—to get all of their good feelings about themselves—through their appearance. It's evident how women are socialized to "use" their appearance to attract others (males) to further define themselves as Somebody's Girlfriend, Somebody's Wife—at a cost to their identities and to themselves.

Recovered women also know that by concentrating their energies on simply being themselves — pursuing their passions and what they love — this intense preoccupation with cultivating and perfecting their appearances will fall by the wayside. There's no use for it anymore, because what they're doing and expressing is so much more meaningful.

"It's life!" Helena exclaims. "It's not looking just at yourself. Suddenly, you can look out and see other people. My eyes are more open now. I feel that I love people. I love people! I love to be alive! The center of my life is to work and think and look and feel that I am doing the best thing that I can with my life. I want to do something *good* with it — something meaningful, something responsible, and not be caught up in the rat race. It's so easy to go around and around in the circles that society sets up for us. Many people have emptiness in their lives, I think because there are so many demands everywhere. I love my work, but I know of other people who work in factories. They just come in, they do their work, they go home, they look at the television, and then they are thinking about the weeks in the summertime when they have their vacations. And that's all they live for. I think it's so important for everyone to have happiness every day, to do something they love. You can't have happiness all the time, but you *can* feel that you are alive in the moment."

In Helena's case, returning to her spiritual faith has been extremely important in her search for meaning. "In the beginning of my teenage years, I had faith in God," Helena says, "and then during my anorexia, I had no time and no interest. I just thought that I didn't want to be at all. Me and my person, I stuck away somewhere, and all other people meant something, but I didn't mean anything at all. But now, I have a faith. I believe that all the things I am doing have meaning for me. With everything I have gone through, I have grown in ways that I needed, that you need in the world. Sometimes things happen, and you can say that it's so cruel, but I think there's meaning in everything. Sometimes, with accidents, you cannot understand why, but there is meaning. I don't know — perhaps the meaning is that you cannot understand everything. And perhaps some people have to get awakened through anorexia to understand that life is not just 'food, food, food.'"

In time, when the distance between anorexia nervosa and the recovered woman is farther and farther away, she'll appreciate the remarkable difference between the woman she was and the woman she has become. She'll be startled to realize that now she *knows* what it means to be happy, pursue her dreams and do what she loves.

Suddenly, she'll marvel and wonder how she ever lived as she did — believing that thinness, weight and calories were the only things that meant anything in life. When she looks back at the "old self," she'll feel love and compassion because she'll know she was coping the only way she knew how.

The recovered anorexic will feel proud of what she has gone through, proud of the battle waged and won, because she has grown so much in her journey to recover. Anorexia nervosa is part of who she is. It has shaped the woman she has become and has made her strong. Because of that experience, she can cope more effectively with the challenges life has in store for her, because she is a survivor. She beat anorexia nervosa. The hard part is over and the only thing she needs to do now is simply be herself.

Finally, she is free.

Reference Notes

Introduction

1. American Psychiatric Association, *Diagnostic and Statistical Manual of Mental Disorders, Third Edition — Revised* (Washington, DC: American Psychiatric Association, 1987).

Chapter 1

1. Paul E. Garfinkel and David M. Garner, *Anorexia Nervosa: A Multidimensional Perspective* (New York: Brunner/Mazel, 1982).

2. Donald M. Schwartz, Michael G. Thompson, and Craig L. Johnson, "Anorexia Nervosa and Bulimia: The Socio-Cultural Context," *International Journal of Eating Disorders*, Spring 1982.

3. Linda Tschirhart Sanford and Mary Ellen Donovan, *Women & Self-Esteem* (New York: Penguin, 1985), pp. xiv-xv.

Chapter 2

1. Susan Wooley and Orland Wooley, "Obesity and Women — I. A Closer Look at the Facts," *Women's Studies International Quarterly*, Summer 1979.

2. Paul E. Garfinkel and David M. Garner, *Anorexia Nervosa: A Multidimensional Perspective* (New York: Brunner/Mazel, 1982), p. 106.

3. Susie Orbach, *Hunger Strike* (New York: Norton, 1986), p. 126.

4. Marlene Boskind-White, "Bulimarexia: A Sociocultural Perspective," ed. Steven Wiley Emmett, *Theory and Treatment of Anorexia Nervosa and Bulimia: Biomedical, Sociocultural, and Psychological Perspectives* (New York: Brunner/Mazel, 1985), p. 114.

5. Garfinkel and Garner, op. cit., p. 111.

6. Ibid., pp. 107-112.

7. Hilde Bruch, *The Golden Cage: The Enigma of Anorexia Nervosa* (New York: Vintage, 1979), p. viii.

8. Richard A. Gordon, *Anorexia and Bulimia: Anatomy of a Social Epidemic* (Cambridge, MA: Basil Blackwell, 1990), pp. 40-1.

9. Felicia F. Romeo, "Anorexia Nervosa: Sociological Considerations for the Private Practitioner," *Psychotherapy in Private Practice*, Fall 1983.

10. Gordon, op. cit., pp. 62-3.

Chapter 3

1. W. Nicholson Browning, "Long-Term Dynamic Group Therapy with Bulimic Patients: A Clinical Discussion," ed. Steven Wiley Emmett, *Theory and Treatment of Anorexia Nervosa and Bulimia: Biomedical, Sociocultural, and Psychological Perspectives*, (New York: Brunner/Mazel, 1985).

2. Donald W. Schwartz, Michael G. Thompson, and Craig L. Johnson, "Anorexia Nervosa and Bulimia: The Socio-Cultural Context," *International Journal of Eating Disorders*, Spring 1982.

Chapter 4

1. Carol Poston and Karen Lison, *Reclaiming Our Lives: Hope for Adult Survivors of Incest* (Boston: Little Brown and Company, 1989).

2. Linda Tschirhart Sanford and Mary Ellen Donovan, *Women & Self-Esteem* (New York: Penguin, 1985), p. 199.

3. Hilde Bruch, *Eating Disorders: Obesity, Anorexia Nervosa, and the Person Within* (New York: Basic Books, 1973), p. 101.

Chapter 5

1. Felicia Romeo, *Understanding Anorexia Nervosa* (Springfield, IL: Charles C Thomas, 1986), pp. 54-5.

2. Michele Siegel, Judith Brisman, and Margot Weinshel, *Surviving an Eating Disorder*, (New York: Harper & Row, 1988), p. 116.

Chapter 7

1. Marion Woodman, *Addiction to Perfection: The Still Unravished Bride* (Toronto: Inner City Books, 1982), p. 19.

Chapter 8

1. Susie Orbach, *Fat Is a Feminist Issue*, (New York: Paddington Press, 1978).

2. Linda Tschirhart Sanford & Mary Ellen Donovan, *Women & Self-Esteem*, (New York: Penguin, 1985), p. 381.

3. Abraham H. Maslow, *The Farther Reaches of Human Nature* (New York: Viking, 1971), pp. 301-2.

4. Viktor E. Frankl, *The Unheard Cry for Meaning* (New York: Washington Square Press, 1978), p. 43.

Resources

American Anorexia/Bulimia Association, Inc. (AABA)
418 East 76th Street
New York, NY 10021
(212) 734-1114

AABA is a tax-exempt, non-profit organization that provides information on self-help/support groups, counseling referrals, and publishes a quarterly newsletter. Through the AABA Recovery Bureau, you may correspond with or talk to other women who have recovered from anorexia nervosa. Membership fees are $50/yr., or for the newsletter only, $40/yr. Write or call for more information.

Anorexia Bulimia Care, Inc. (ABC)
P.O. Box 213
Lincoln Center, MA 01773
(617) 259-9767

ABC sponsors support groups throughout Massachusetts and offers lectures and referrals throughout New England. Membership fees are $25/yr. for individuals, $50/yr. for professionals and families, and $50 for organizations. Send $1 and a self-addressed, stamped envelope for more information.

Anorexia Nervosa and Related Eating Disorders, Inc. (ANRED)
P.O. Box 5102
Eugene, OR 97405
(503) 344-1144

ANRED is a membership-supported organization that publishes a four-page newsletter, *ANRED Alert*, ten times a year, offers information on treatment programs, sells booklets and brochures, and sponsors support groups in the Eugene, Oregon area. Membership fees are $10/yr. Write or call for more information.

National Anorexic Aid Society (NAAS)
1925 East Dublin-Granville Road
Columbus, OH 43229-3517
(614) 436-1112

NAAS publishes a quarterly newsletter (January, April, July, and October), offers support groups in the Central Ohio area, provides information, referrals, educational programs, counselor training, and sponsors a national conference each fall. Annual membership fees are $12 for students, $20 for individuals and families, and $35 for organizations. Send a $5 check or money order for an eating disorder information packet.

National Association of Anorexia Nervosa
and Associated Disorders (ANAD)
Box 7
Highland Park, IL 60035
(708) 831-3438

ANAD offers many free services, including counseling, information referrals, self-help groups for anorexics and their families, education programs, and a listing of therapists, hospitals, and clinics treating eating disorders. Membership fees are $25/yr. Send $1 for a packet of information.

Anorexics/Bulimics Anonymous (ABA)
P.O. Box 178414
San Diego, CA 92177
(619) 273-3108

ABA is a twelve-step program for anyone who wishes to recover from anorexia nervosa and/or bulimia. Their program differs from Overeaters Anonymous in that they do not include the concept of "abstinence" in recovery. ABA sponsors meetings in the San Diego area and offers information on how to start support groups. There are no membership fees. Call or write for a packet of information.

Index

Achievement mandates, 37-39,
    46-49
Amenorrhea, 3,5,20
Anorexia nervosa
    acceleration of, 61-67
    admitting, 83-87,92-93,96-97,119
    as a coping strategy, 18-19,22,
        60-61,71
    as an addiction, 21,23,62-63,80
    as an escape, 39,66,71
    clinical definition of, 5
    communicating through,
        69-71,97,101-102
    exploring underlying issues of,
        95-103,106-107
    identifying the self with,
        61-62,66,69-70
    multi-determined causes, 21-22
    onset of, 1-2,28,55-67; *see also*
        Triggering factors
    surge in reported cases, 32,35,53
    underlying messages of, 10-11,
        69-72,98-99; *see also*
        Symbolism
Appearance
    defining oneself through, 30-32,
        37,71,121-123,133
    losing preoccupation with, 134
    rejecting emphasis on, 122-126

Beauty ideals, 25-27,29-30,36-37,
    121-123
    ever-changing, 32-33,122
    rejecting, 121-126
Binging, 60,74,117
Body image distortions, 2-3,5,24,31,
    56,63
    changing, 98,117

Body insecurity, 30-31,33-34,123,
    125
Boskind-White, Marlene, 31
Brisman, Judith, 81
Browning, W. Nicholson, 50
Bruch, Hilde, 35,62

Carpenter, Karen, 35
Cognitive distortions, 11-13,63-64;
    see also Body image distortions,
    Denial, Emptiness
Comparison to others, 12,34
    competition, 16,29,80-82
    preoccupation with others'
        opinions, 14; *see also*
        People-pleasing
    siblings, 47-48
Conditional love, 46-54
Control
    fear of losing, 13,72,76-77,95
    food as, 17,72,99
    illusion of anorexia nervosa as,
        83-84
    in recovery, 110-111
    letting go of, 96,103,106
    over one's life, 19-24,55,58-61

Deception, 13-14,72-76
Denial
    breaking through the, 86-87,92-93,
        96-97,119
    of anorexia nervosa, 2,5,36,62-64,
        72-75,80,85,101
    of hunger, 10,62
Diet pills, 2,73
Donovan, Mary Ellen, 22,59,124

Eating
   discomfort about, 14,87,115-116
   normal patterns of, 17-18,117-121
Emptiness, 9-24,105,127,134
   at the center of one's existence, 17
   attempting to fill the, 24,87,116
   symbolic representations of, 10,85

False self, 49-51
Families, 41-54
   dysfunctional, 18
   exasperation of, 12-13
   perceived as conditionally loving,
      46-54
   strengthening relationships within,
      130-131
   trying to please, 46-47,50-51,
      53-54
   valuing thinness, 41-46
Fashion models, 25,30,33-34
Fat
   fear of, 5,27,97-98
   oppression, 28,33,43-44,55
Feelings
   acceptance of, 89,103
   blocking, 71-72,98
   confusion over, 17,21,99
   denial of, 66,71-72
   getting in touch with, 98-105
   numbing, 39,98-99,105
   of anger, 98,104-105
   of superiority, 3,63-64
   working through, 110-111
Frankl, Viktor, 128-129

Garfinkel, Paul E., 21,29-30,31,33
Garner, David M., 21,29-30,31,33
Gordon, Richard A., 37,38-39
Group meetings
   pitfalls of, 80-82
   in recovery, 91-94,100

Health care professionals. *See also*
      Therapy
   deceiving, 13-14,72-75
Health spas, 1-2
Hospitalization
   in life-threatening situations, 6,76,
      95
   shortcomings of, 74-80,84
   benefits of long-term treatment
      programs, 3,76-78
Hunger
   denial of, 10,62
   responding to, 119-120

Identity issues, 61-62,66,69-70,
      103,133. *See also* False self

Johnson, Craig L., 21,53

Malibu Barbie, 26,38
Madonna, 27,30
Male approval, 29,33,42
   Fathers, 46-47
Maslow, Abraham, 127
Meaning, 127-135
Media messages, 25-35,60
   confused, 38
   glamorizing anorexia nervosa,
      35-36
   rejecting, 122-125
   see also Societal messages
Miss America pageant contestants,
      33
Mother-bashing, 51,53

Objectification of women, 25-31. *See
   also* Beauty ideals
Obsessional behavior, 24,62,71-74,
      83-84; *see also* Emptiness,
      Control
   calorie-counting, 10,14,20,64-65
   compulsive activity, 19-21

disturbed eating patterns, 9-11,
65-66
hyperexercising, 15-16,79
rigid weight control, 19-20
Onset, 1-2,55-67. *See also* Triggering
factors
Orbach, Susie, 30,119
Overeaters Anonymous, 93-94,120

Passion, 127-128
Peer pressure, 28-29,44,55
People-pleasing, 50-51,53-54. *See
also* Male approval
Perfection
in appearance, 19,34; *see also*
Beauty ideals
letting go of, 108-109,111,126
perceived expectations of, 49
unrealistic ideals of, 11,16,22-23,
50-54,102-103
Personal relationships
fear of, 66,90-91,105-106
in recovery, 4,87-88,108,112,
125-126,132-133
isolation, 19,66-67
loss of, 57-58
through support groups, 91-94
Playboy Playmate of the Month, 33

Recovery
as a process, 100-101,106-108,
113,115-135
changing behaviors, 116-117,
121
choices in, 76,85-86,113,119
first step toward, 86-87
hitting bottom, 84-85
resistance to, 69-70,72-77; *see
also* Denial
spiritual faith in, 134
strategies in, 98-100,110-113,
129-135
support groups in, 91-94
therapy in, 88-90,99

Research methodology, 6-7
Role models, 26-27
Romeo, Felicia, 37,77

Sanford, Linda Tschirhart, 22,59,124
Schwartz, Donald M., 21,53
Seigel, Michele, 81
Self-acceptance, 4-5,107,123-127
Self-actualization. *See* Meaning
Self-assertion, 4,90,102-106,126,
131-132
lack of, 3
Self-esteem
in recovery, 22,124
low, 19,22-23,33,53-54,107
Self-exploration, 4,99,102-103,
106-107,127
Self-hatred, 33,84-85,98,122
Self-love, 4-5,94,107
Self-punishment, 11
Self-worth, 131-132
lack of, 12,23,84
Sex role stereotypes, 25-26
Sexual abuse, 52,55,71,96
Sexual harassment, 3
Slim-Fast, 28
Societal messages
contradictory, 15,38
dieting as achievement, 3,23,31
of thinness, 17,25-35,123
pressure to achieve, 37-39,46-49
regarding appearance,
25-26,71,133; *see also*
Appearance, Beauty ideals
rejecting, 122-125
Standards of beauty. *See* Beauty
ideals, Appearance
Superwoman ideals,
37-39,49,60,102-103
Support groups, 91-94
Overeaters Anonymous, 93-94,120
see also Group meetings
Symbolism
of anorexia nervosa, 10-11,69-72,
98-99

of thinness, 11,23,29-30,43,55
of weight as protection, 4

Therapy
  in recovery, 88-90,99
Thinness
  and attractiveness, 29-30,32
  valuation of, 35-37,41-46
  symbolism of, 11,23,29-30,43,
    55,69-72
  see also Appearance, Beauty
    ideals
Thompson, Michael G., 21,53
Triggering factors, 22,55-60
  break-up of relationships, 57-58
  craving attention, 52-53,
    56-57
  geographical move, 57
  job pressures, 58-60
  losing a best friend, 56
  marriage, 58
  rape, 58-59

sexual abuse, 52-55
starting college, 1-2
taunting from peers, 28-29,44,55
Trust
  in recovery, 90,97-98,101-102

Unconditional acceptance, 4,87-90

Vomiting, 20,74

Weight gain
  fear of, 5,16,95-96,115-116
  accepting, 124
  resistance to, 15,97,116
Weinshel, Margot, 81
Western values, 37,46
Women's magazines, 31,33-35,44
  rejecting messages of, 124-125
Woodman, Marion, 103
Wooley, Susan and Orland, 28